# Staying Flexible
*The Full Range of Motion*

*Fitness, Health & Nutrition* was created by Rebus, Inc. and published by Time-Life Books.

## REBUS, INC.

Publisher: RODNEY FRIEDMAN

Editor: CHARLES L. MEE JR.
Senior Editor: THOMAS DICKEY
Managing Editor: SUSAN BRONSON
Senior Writer: WILLIAM DUNNETT
Associate Editors: NONA CLELAND, CARL LOWE
Contributing Editor: PAUL PERRY

Art Director: ROBBIN SCHIFF
Designer: DEBORAH RAGASTO
Photographer: STEVEN MAYS
Photo Stylist: NOLA LOPEZ

Recipe Editor: BONNIE J. SLOTNICK
Contributing Editor, Food: MARYA DALRYMPLE
Test Kitchen Director: ANNE DISRUDE
Consulting Editor, Food: SALLY SCHNEIDER
Nutritional Analyst: HILL NUTRITION ASSOCIATES

Chief of Research: CARNEY W. MIMMS III
Assistant Editor: JACQUELINE DILLON

Time-Life Books Inc. is a wholly owned subsidiary of
**TIME INCORPORATED**

Founder: HENRY R. LUCE 1898-1967

Editor-in-Chief: HENRY ANATOLE GRUNWALD
Chairman and Chief Executive Officer: J. RICHARD MUNRO
President and Chief Operating Officer: N.J. NICHOLAS JR.
Chairman of the Executive Committee: RALPH P. DAVIDSON
Corporate Editor: RAY CAVE
Executive Vice President, Books: KELSO F. SUTTON
Vice President, Books: GEORGE ARTANDI

## TIME-LIFE BOOKS INC.

Editor: GEORGE CONSTABLE

Director of Design: LOUIS KLEIN
Director of Editorial Resources: PHYLLIS K. WISE
Acting Text Director: ELLEN PHILLIPS
Editorial Board: RUSSELL B. ADAMS JR., DALE M. BROWN, ROBERTA CONLAN, THOMAS H. FLAHERTY, DONIA ANN STEELE, ROSALIND STUBENBERG, KIT VAN TULLEKEN, HENRY WOODHEAD
Director of Photography and Research: JOHN CONRAD WEISER

President: CHRISTOPHER T. LINEN
Executive Vice President: JOHN M. FAHEY JR.
Senior Vice Presidents: JAMES L. MERCER, LEOPOLDO TORALBALLA
Vice Presidents: STEPHEN L. BAIR, RALPH J. CUOMO, TERENCE J. FURLONG, NEAL GOFF, STEPHEN L. GOLDSTEIN, JUANITA T. JAMES, HALLETT JOHNSON III, ROBERT H. SMITH, PAUL R. STEWART
Director of Production Services: ROBERT J. PASSANTINO

*Editorial Operations*
Copy Chief: DIANE ULLIUS
Editorial Operations: CAROLINE A. BOUBIN (MANAGER)
Production: CELIA BEATTIE
Quality Control: JAMES J. COX (DIRECTOR)
Library: LOUISE D. FORSTALL

FITNESS, HEALTH & NUTRITION

# Staying Flexible
## *The Full Range of Motion*

*Time-Life Books, Alexandria, Virginia*

## CONSULTANTS FOR THIS BOOK

Charles B. Corbin, Ph.D., is Professor in the Department of Health and Physical Education at Arizona State University, Tempe. He is the author of several books, including *Concepts of Physical Fitness* and *Fitness for Life*, and has written numerous articles for scholarly journals. Dr. Corbin was honored as a Prince Philip Lecturer by the British Physical Education Association and is a Fellow of the American Academy of Physical Education.

Risa Friedman holds a master's degree in dance education and is certified in health fitness by the American College of Sports Medicine, the International Dance Exercise Association and the Laban-Bartenieff Institute of Movement Studies. She has taught anatomy/kinesiology, movement analysis, therapeutic exercise, exercise physiology, and fitness and dance at New York University and the State University of New York, among other institutions. She is currently an exercise physiologist in private practice in San Diego, California, and is Program Director of the Fitness Specialist Certification Program at Marymount Manhattan College in New York City.

Judy L. Marriott is a Certified Movement Analyst with the Laban-Bartenieff Institute of Movement Studies and has worked as an exercise trainer since 1984. She is also a professional dancer and has performed with several companies nationally and internationally.

Marika E. Molnar is a physical therapist for the New York City Ballet. She is also a director at a Manhattan sports medicine center and has lectured and written about the prevention and rehabilitation of dance injuries.

Myron Winick, M.D., is the R.R. Williams Professor of Nutrition, Professor of Pediatrics, Director of the Institute of Human Nutrition, and Director of the Center for Nutrition, Genetics and Human Development at Columbia University College of Physicians and Surgeons. He has served on the Food and Nutrition Board of the National Academy of Sciences and is the author of many books, including *Your Personalized Health Profile*.

For information about any Time-Life book please write:
Reader Information
Time-Life Books
541 North Fairbanks Court
Chicago
Illinois 60611

First printing.
Published simultaneously in Canada.
School and library distribution by Silver Burdett Company, Morristown, New Jersey.

TIME-LIFE is a trademark of Time Incorporated U.S.A.

Library of Congress Cataloging-in-Publication Data
Getting firm.
Includes index.
1. Physical fitness. 2. Exercise. I. Time-Life Books. II. Series
GV481.S718 1987 613.7'1 86-30099
ISBN 0-8094-6167-6
ISBN 0-8094-6168-4 (lib. bdg.)

This book is not intended as a substitute for the advice of a physician. Readers who have, or suspect they may have, specific medical problems, especially those involving their muscles and joints, are urged to consult a physician before beginning any program of strenuous physical exercise.

# CONTENTS

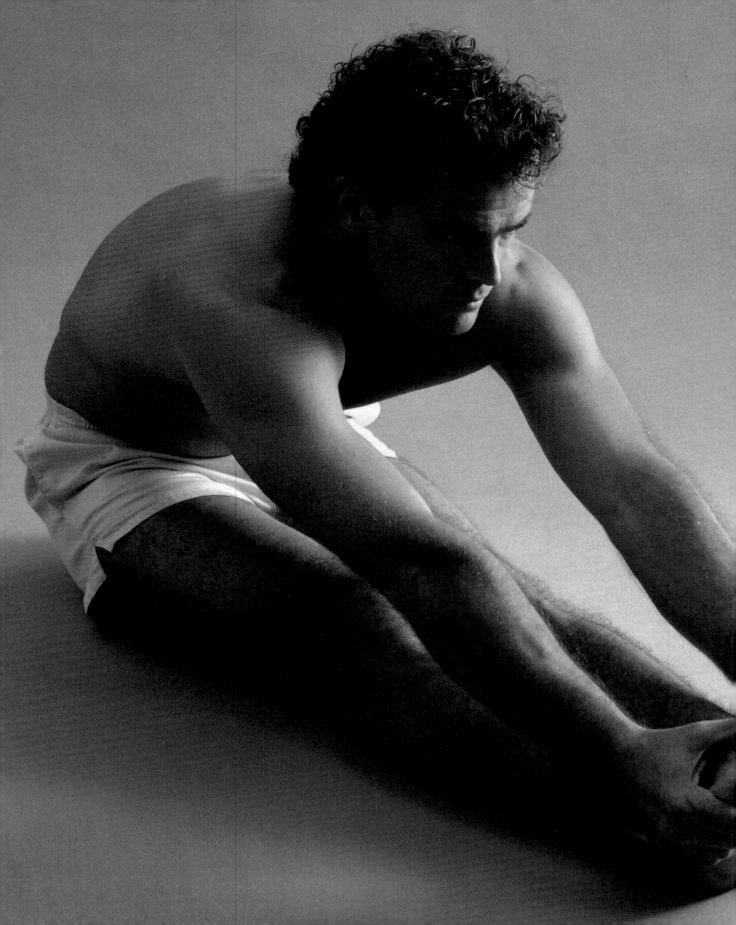

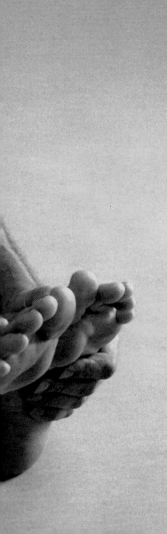

# CHAPTER ONE

# Flexibility

*Lengthening muscles
with the right stretches for
greater agility, better posture and
insurance against injury*

Physical fitness is more than just endurance or muscular strength. It is a complex latticework of many interrelated factors, each important in its own way. One of these factors is flexibility. Perhaps the most neglected aspect of many fitness programs, flexibility training is being increasingly recognized as crucial for complementing muscular strength, building efficiency and coordination, and preventing injuries.

### What is flexibility?
Flexibility is the mobility or range of motion in a joint. This range of motion is determined by the natural structure of the joint itself and the direction in which it bends. Ball-and-socket joints, such as those in your hips and shoulders, afford greater range of motion than the hinge joints in your knees and elbows, the condyloid joints in your wrists, the pivot joints in your spinal column or the gliding joints in the metatarsals of your feet.

## Improving Flexibility

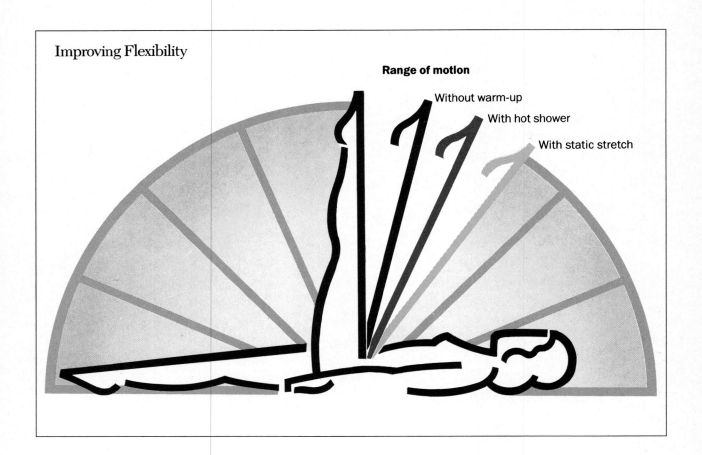

**Range of motion**

Without warm-up

With hot shower

With static stretch

A five-minute shower under hot water (109-113° F) will increase the flexibility of your hip joint so that it can move five percent farther than it can when you are not warmed up. Static stretching can increase your range of motion another two to four percent.

A joint is flexible when the muscles and connective tissues around it do not restrict its natural range of motion. You should, for example, be able to extend your arm straight out at a 90-degree angle from your body and then flex your elbow joint enough to rest your hand comfortably on your shoulder. A flexible elbow joint allows full extension and flexion of your arm.

### What limits flexibility?

When a joint moves, resistance from soft tissue is the major obstacle to its full natural range of movement. Researchers have determined that skin provides two percent of that resistance, tendons and ligaments 10 percent, and muscle tissue and its connecting fascia, 41 percent. The remaining resistance is in the joint capsule itself. Since the joint capsule, tendons and ligaments are composed of collagen, a nonelastic connective tissue, the length of muscles — which are both elastic and extensible — is usually the determining factor in the joint's range of motion. A "short" muscle limits range of motion; a "long" muscle allows a full, natural range of motion.

### Are some people naturally more flexible than others?

Yes, but there is no ideal or standard for flexibility. The only standards available are based on norms that indicate how hundreds of individuals of both sexes and various age groups have performed. Generally speaking, tests have shown that children are more flexible than adults and that women are more flexible than men. Two studies, for instance, tested the flexibility of 510 males aged 18 to 71 and 407 females aged 18 to 74. These studies found that, for the average man tested, flexibility was greatest for most muscle groups and joints between the ages of 23 and 24; among women, it was greatest between the ages of 25 and 29.

Another study measured the flexibility of 300 randomly selected girls between the ages of six and 18. In most of the 12 flexibility measurements the researchers took, the girls' flexibility increased from age six to age 12 and then showed a decline. But the results were inconsistent: In terms of shoulder, knee and hip flexibility, there was a decrease between the ages of six and 18; yet 18-year-olds were more flexible in their trunk and wrist muscles and had better flexibility in the muscles along the outside of their thighs than younger girls.

### Is there a simple way to test flexibility?

For a long time, it was thought that flexibility was a general characteristic of the body: You were either flexible or you were not. However, researchers have now determined that flexibility is not equally apparent in all joints of the body. Just as there is a great range of flexibility among individuals in the same age and sex group, studies show that flexibility can even change drastically from one muscle group to another. In the study of 300 girls cited above, for instance, no girl was above or below average in all measurements of flexibility. You can have tight hamstrings and supple shoulder muscles, or tight hip flexors but flexible trunk muscles. You can even have bilateral differences in flexibility — your right quadriceps, for example, can be less flexible than your left.

Flexibility in a joint also changes according to the direction in which the joint moves. You can be quite flexible when you bend your arm in one direction, for example, but less flexible when you use different muscles to rotate your arm in another direction. Also, the relation of one joint to another may influence the range of motion in one or both joints. For instance, if you are like most people, you can easily flex your fingers and tuck them into the palm of your hand so long as your wrist is extended. But if you flex your wrist, you will significantly reduce the range of motion in your finger joints, and you may not be able to tuck your fingers into your palm.

Clearly, flexibility is highly specific, making it difficult to provide an overall measurement without testing virtually every joint in the body. But you can get a general idea of your level of flexibility by taking several key measurements. The tests on pages 18-19 will help you define your own level of flexibility.

### Why is staying flexible important?

For the athletic person, most experts believe that good flexibility

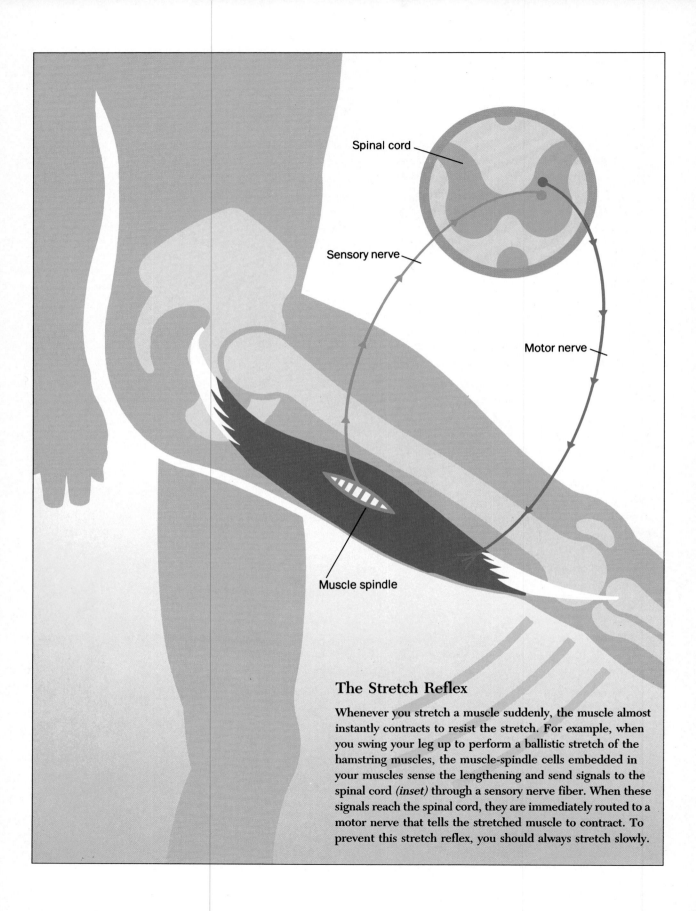

Spinal cord

Sensory nerve

Motor nerve

Muscle spindle

## The Stretch Reflex

Whenever you stretch a muscle suddenly, the muscle almost instantly contracts to resist the stretch. For example, when you swing your leg up to perform a ballistic stretch of the hamstring muscles, the muscle-spindle cells embedded in your muscles sense the lengthening and send signals to the spinal cord *(inset)* through a sensory nerve fiber. When these signals reach the spinal cord, they are immediately routed to a motor nerve that tells the stretched muscle to contract. To prevent this stretch reflex, you should always stretch slowly.

reduces the chance of injury. Muscles that are short and restrict the natural range of motion in the joints are more susceptible to pulls, tears and stress injuries than those that are long enough to allow a full range of motion. Good flexibility also improves athletic performance. Short muscles detract from the grace of the gymnast, dancer and ice skater, may limit the muscular power of the golfer and tennis and baseball player, and may even lead to injury. Short calf muscles, for instance, can place undue stress on the foot, leading to a variety of orthopedic problems, including painful Achilles tendinitis.

Flexibility is also crucial for proper posture, which in turn affects both your athletic performance and your general well-being. Persons who stand and sit correctly — their head centered, shoulders down and back, chest high and abdomen flat — give the impression of being alert and confident. Those who slump and have rounded shoulders, drooping head and excessive curvature of the spine — due to short chest, hamstring and pelvic muscles — may develop a poor self-image and convey an unfavorable impression to others.

### Can a lack of flexibility cause health problems?

Lack of flexibility can create poor posture, resulting in mechanical imbalances in the back, hip and neck. These imbalances pull body segments out of line, causing stress, strain and even worse posture. The resulting muscular tension, joint strain and ligament and cartilage damage can produce deformity. Short chest muscles and weak shoulders, for instance, cause rounded shoulders, which can lead to kyphosis (humpbacked spine), a sunken chest and impaired respiratory capacity. Tight hip-flexor muscles, short hamstrings and back muscles can rotate the pelvis forward, resulting in lordosis (excessive curvature of the lower back), chronic lower back pain and sciatica (a radiating pain in the thighs or buttocks along the sciatic nerve). Drooping your head forward may produce headache, dizziness and chronic strain on the muscles along the back of the neck, resulting in neck and shoulder pain.

### How can you increase your flexibility?

Simply using your muscles will help lengthen them to some extent. For instance, you are usually the least flexible when you get out of bed in the morning. Then, just by engaging in your normal routine and using your muscles to walk, sit and stand, you gradually gain flexibility throughout the day. The vigorous movement of exercise also helps: Studies show that calisthenics, for example, increase flexibility. In general, athletes and people who work out regularly are more flexible than nonathletes and sedentary persons.

You can even increase flexibility, however slightly, by taking a hot shower (see illustration page 8). Warming connective tissue appears to increase its pliability: One study showed that by deep-tissue warming to 113° F, you can increase the range of motion in a joint by as much as 20 percent. Cooling the joint to 65° F reduces flexibility by 10 to 20 percent. These changes in flexibility are temporary, however. The

## Stretch to Run

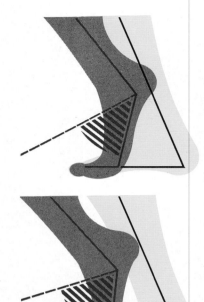

Flexible calf muscles and ankles help you run better. The farther the muscles and tendons of your calf, ankle and foot are stretched, the longer your foot stays in contact with the ground, letting you push off harder with each running step you take.

preferred method of enhancing muscular flexibility is through a stretching program.

### Can a muscle stretch itself?

Muscles are like ropes: They exert force by pulling, not pushing. Similarly, muscles cannot lengthen themselves; they can only contract and relax. Most skeletal muscles are attached to one or more joints. When they contract, they move the joints. Therefore, stretching a muscle requires an external force, such as gravity or the contraction of an opposing muscle, to move a joint and stretch the muscle. Each of the exercises in this book uses such a force to achieve a stretch.

### How much stretching is required to make a muscle more flexible?

To increase a muscle's length, studies show, you must regularly pull it about 10 percent beyond its normal length: That is the point where your muscle feels stretched enough to be slightly uncomfortable but not enough to cause pain.

### How often should you stretch?

The idea of lengthening a muscle in a progressive stretching program to increase flexibility is related to the overload principle used to build muscle strength. To increase muscular strength, you must regularly contract the muscle against resistance with a slightly greater force than it is used to. In time, the muscle responds to the overload by becoming stronger. Similarly, to increase flexibility, you must regularly stretch the muscle slightly beyond its normal length. It will adapt to this overload by becoming longer, rewarding you with a greater range of joint motion. Studies show that you should stretch three to seven days a week to increase your flexibility. For maintaining flexibility, three days a week is probably adequate.

### What are some of the immediate benefits of stretching?

Stretching is a natural, relaxing sensation. It helps relieve tension and the feeling of stiffness. Many people stretch in one way or another right after getting out of bed in the morning. Most people also stretch intermittently while sitting at a desk or driving a car for long periods. These simple routines do not increase general or long-term flexibility — they are simply pleasurable movements.

Stretching is not only pleasurable, it can also alleviate pain. For example, since one common cause of lower back pain is short, tight hip-flexor muscles, a stretching program to lengthen these muscles may reduce the risk of lower back pain. Some experts think that stretching can help prevent or alleviate about 80 percent of all cases of lower back pain; that 80 percent is caused by tightness and spasms in the musculature of the back and pelvis.

You can also stretch to reduce muscle soreness associated with stress injuries, which result from overdoing sports and exercise. According to one theory, this type of soreness is produced by a cycle of

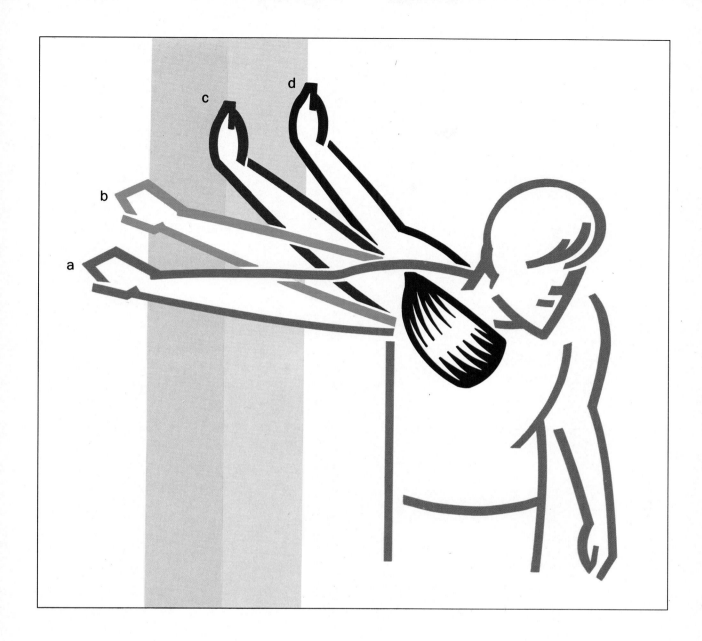

## Four Types of Stretches

Not all stretching techniques are equally able to lengthen muscles. Say, for example, you want to stretch your chest muscle, which you use to swing your arm forward. By swiftly swinging your arm backward, the momentum forces the chest muscle to stretch. But this sudden ballistic movement induces the stretch reflex *(see illustration page 10)*, and your chest muscle contracts. As a result, a ballistic stretch allows

your arm to swing only about 90 degrees (a). You can override the stretch reflex by swinging your arm back slowly. This sustained, or static, stretch increases the range of motion by a few more degrees (b).

You can increase a static stretch by using an external force, such as someone pushing your arm back, or by holding your hand against a wall and turning your body against the stretch

(c). Most of the stretches in Chapters Two and Four rely on this technique. The longest stretch of all (d) is possible with a method called contract-relax, explained in Chapter Three. This technique entails briefly contracting the muscle to be stretched while a partner, a wall or any other external force prevents movement. As you relax, your limb can be pushed into an even greater stretch.

muscle tension, soreness and increased neural reflex activity, which results in more muscle tension and soreness. Slow, deliberate stretching reduces the neural activity in the muscles, thus breaking the cycle and reducing the pain.

**What is the difference between a flexibility training program and using stretches to warm up?**
A flexibility training program consists of stretching exercises designed to improve general flexibility when performed regularly. These exercises should work on muscle groups all over the body, concentrating on the tighter muscles. A flexibility warm-up is a group of stretches performed just before engaging in exercise or sports and is designed to temporarily elongate the muscles directly involved in that activity. For instance, stretching out for running would involve working primarily on the hip flexors, quadriceps, hamstrings and calves. The warm-up routine is less extensive than the flexibility training program and therefore less effective for improving general long-term flexibility. There is no evidence to suggest that sporadic flexibility warm-ups can result in long-term gains in joint range of motion such as those attained by a regular flexibility training program. Stretching exercises as part of a sports warm-up, however, have been shown to increase a joint's range of motion by four to 18 percent for 90 minutes or more. For more information on stretching routines designed for specific sports, turn to Chapter Four.

**Is it dangerous to have too much flexibility?**
Too much flexibility without muscle strength can cause instability in the joints, leading to dislocations and other traumas. Victims of poliomyelitis and other diseases or injuries of the neuromuscular system may suffer from this condition. However, it is unlikely that you can ever become so flexible from a stretching program that you will have this problem. Nor will you become "double-jointed," a congenital condition that results in unusually flexible joints and permits contortions of limbs and torso.

Overly flexible or loose joints can result from stretching ligaments, the connective tissue that binds joints together. Ligaments, unlike muscles, are not elastic and therefore remain lengthened when stretched repeatedly. Weight-bearing joints such as the knee, ankle or hip may become unstable and susceptible to dislocation or abnormal twisting, resulting in injury. It is widely accepted among athletes that loose joints can lead to injury; many athletes therefore tape joints to increase stability. Most athletes who have loose joints also strengthen the supporting muscles in order to improve control over their joint flexibility. Their concern may be unwarranted, however, since studies do not show a direct correlation between loose joints and frequency of athletic injuries.

*S tudies show that stretching can help relieve delayed muscle soreness after strenuous exercise. And evidence now suggests that stretching can at least reduce and sometimes prevent dysmenorrhea, or painful menstruation. If you suffer from dysmenorrhea that is not the result of a disease, you can probably relieve your symptoms by regularly performing stretching exercises of the muscles in the pelvic region.*

### Does weight training reduce flexibility?

Although it is commonly thought that musclebound people are inflexible, studies show that strength training, when done properly, does not limit flexibility. Body builders who regularly stretch their muscles as well as strengthen them have better-than-average flexibility.

### What are the most important muscles to stretch?

Since flexibility is specific, you can increase a muscle's length only by stretching that particular muscle. Studies show, however, that people who stretch tend to stretch their longest muscles and neglect their shortest. The problem, then, is to identify the muscles that are tight and spend the bulk of your stretching time working on them, not on muscles that are already sufficiently flexible.

Generally speaking, the muscles most in need of stretching are the ones on which you place the greatest demands. Most reasonably active people should routinely stretch the following muscles: calves (to increase the range of motion in ankles and to prevent calf pain and Achilles tendinitis), hamstrings (to prevent running-related injuries), inner thighs (to reduce the chance of groin pulls), quadriceps and hip flexors (to prevent knee stiffness and lower back pain), and chest and shoulders (to prevent rounded shoulders and restricted range of motion).

### Is it ever too late to get flexible?

One of the most obvious signs of advancing age is reduced flexibility. In far too many cases, range of motion becomes so severely restricted that an elderly person may be afraid of getting injured simply by walking or climbing stairs.

Luckily, inflexibility can be reversed, even among the elderly. In a study that compared the joint stiffness of a group of 20 young men (aged 15 to 19) and a group of 20 elderly men (aged 63 to 88), it was found that both groups could reverse joint stiffness with equal ease. A number of other studies have shown that virtually anyone, regardless of age, can improve flexibility by stretching.

I t is widely reported and commonly believed that tall, thin people are generally more flexible than those who are short and stocky. Although studies do suggest a direct relationship of total height and limb length to flexibility, the correlation is so slight that it is of little practical importance.

# How to Design Your Own Program

The simple tests on pages 18-19 will allow you to assess your flexibility. But even before you take the tests, ask yourself the questions here. You do not need to determine your flexibility level precisely — you can often tell how supple your muscles are simply by using them and listening to their signals.

## How flexible are you?

 **Can you touch your toes?**

Touching your toes without bending your knees has been the timeworn test for flexibility. But, in fact, touching your toes tells little more than how flexible you are in the hamstrings and lower back. And, in order to keep you feeling good and safe from injury, flexibility must be a whole-body phenomenon. Some experts believe that the standing toe touch may be dangerous under certain circumstances because it can place stress on the lower back.

 **Can you sit with your legs outstretched and touch your head to your knees?**

Most dancers can, but if you can, you may be trying too hard to become flexible. Forcing a stretch can lengthen ligaments as well as muscles. Muscles have extensibility and elasticity. When you stretch them, they spring back. Ligaments, however, are extensible but not elastic — they will not spring back. Once a ligament is stretched, it will stay stretched and may cause instability in a joint, especially in the hip, knee and ankle. Studies are not conclusive, but it appears that loose ligaments may lead to tears in cartilage and other soft tissue. Never try to force a stretch.

 **Do you often remind yourself to sit up straight and not slump?**

If so, you should probably work on increasing the flexibility in your chest and shoulder muscles so that your posture while sitting and standing is more natural and less stressful.

 **Do you limp around the morning after a strenuous game of tennis or squash?**

If your favorite sport makes you stiff the morning after, you should be working on increasing your flexibility. See Chapter Four for stretching routines specific to eight of the most popular recreational sports.

 **Do you have leg cramps at night?**

These are annoying but harmless. However, they probably indicate that you are overdue for a stretching program. See Chapter Two.

### 6   Do you suffer from backaches frequently?

Backaches are among the nation's major health complaints; yet many of them can be prevented simply by increasing flexibility. Good posture and strong, flexible muscles in the lower back and pelvis may help keep pressure off the disks in the lumbar region and so help prevent the condition that leads to herniated or ruptured disks. The illustration on page 21 will guide you to stretching routines for the back.

### 7   Do you play sports often?

If your answer is yes, then your flexibility may vary depending on the sport you play. Athletes in different sports, studies show, display different flexibility profiles. Baseball and track athletes, for example, outperform wrestlers in certain tests. Furthermore, sports and exercise are selective in the muscles they lengthen. For example, hardly any sport improves the flexibility of inner-thigh muscles, and for athletes these muscles are among the most likely to get torn or pulled, usually from an abrupt lateral leg movement. So if you play sports often, it pays to stretch regularly.

### 8   Do you do ballistic stretches?

That is to say, do you use vigorous bouncing, jerking or rocking movements to stretch your muscles? Since many athletic activities are ballistic in nature, some experts think that some ballistic stretching is good for you after you have already become generally flexible through static stretching exercises. And studies show that ballistic stretching is at least as effective as static stretching for improving flexibility. But there is great potential for pulling or tearing muscles with ballistic stretching, and most people should avoid it altogether.

# Do you get cramps when you work out?

People who engage in sports or other strenuous activities often get muscle cramps. Usually the best way to prevent cramps is by stretching — both before and after exercise. If a cramp does occur, however, the best first aid is to stretch the muscle immediately. Gentle massage also helps.

If the cramp recurs in the same place, it may be a symptom of a slight muscle tear — and a warning to ease up. But sometimes a muscle cramp is brought on by dehydration after prolonged exercise; the dehydration causes an imbalance in calcium, sodium or potassium. If this is the case, there is a simple solution: Drink water before and during exercise. This will usually restore the right mineral balance.

# Measuring Your Flexibility

There is no best level of flexibility for all people. Everyone has a different degree of flexibility that varies from limb to limb, from day to day, sometimes even from hour to hour. No single test can give you a sense of your overall flexibility. However, you can get a general assessment by testing the range of motion you can achieve in the major joints of your body. Furthermore, by taking a number of tests that measure specific muscles and muscle groups, you can determine where to concentrate the most effort.

Perhaps the greatest benefit of a flexibility test is to establish a baseline before beginning your training program. You will then have a gauge by which to measure your progress. The five simple tests on these two pages measure flexibility in the lower back, hamstrings, hip flexors, shoulders and calves — areas where flexibility is particularly important among active people. All you need are a yardstick or ruler and a box or step about eight inches high. Ask a friend to help you take the measurements. Perform the tests about once a month to chart your progress. Remember that you are not in competition with anyone in achieving good flexibility. For the best results in this or any other fitness program, you should proceed at your own pace.

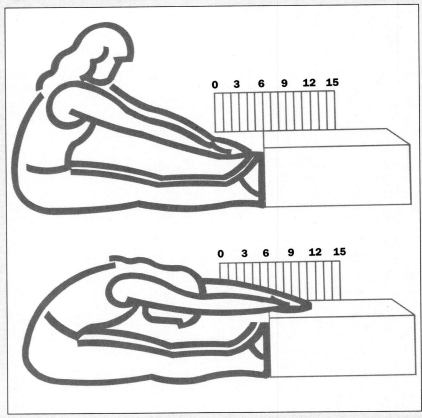

Two of the muscle groups important to your overall flexibility are the lower back and hamstring muscles. To test their flexibility, sit with the soles of your feet against a box or step and your arms outstretched *(top)*. Reach as far forward as you can toward the edge of the box without bending your knees. At the beginning of your flexibility program, you may not be able to reach the box. Later, you may be able to reach as far as the bottom figure. Have a partner record how far your fingertips reach on a yardstick extended six inches in front of the edge of the box. Find your flexibility rating using the chart below.

## How Far Can You Reach?
### (in inches)

|  | **Men** | **Women** |
|---|---|---|
| Excellent | 14+ | 15+ |
| Very good | 11-13 | 12-14 |
| Fair | 7-10 | 7-11 |
| Poor | 4-6 | 4-6 |
| Very poor | 3 or less | 3 or less |

Sit on a box or a straight-backed chair, holding your back erect. Rest one leg on the floor while extending the other. If your hamstrings are adequately flexible, you will be able to extend the leg fully without moving your other leg or altering your upright seated position.

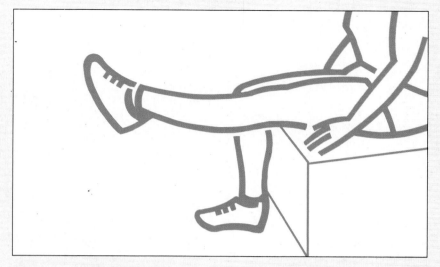

While lying prone with one leg bent, have your partner grasp your knee with one hand and, pushing down on your pelvis with the other, raise your leg. If your quadriceps and hip flexors are flexible, your partner will be able to raise your knee several inches without causing you undue discomfort.

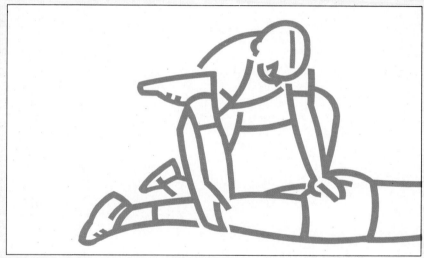

Raise your right elbow and reach behind your back *(near right)*. Place your left hand in the small of your back and slide it upward. If you can touch your hands behind your back and overlap your fingers, your arms and shoulders are adequately flexible. To test your calf muscles, stand about three feet from a wall with your feet spread shoulder-width apart *(far right)*. Place your hands on the wall and bend forward until your chin touches the wall. You should be able to do this while keeping your body straight and your feet flat on the floor.

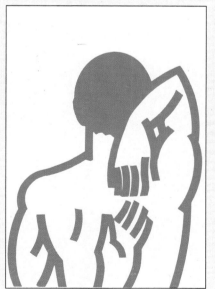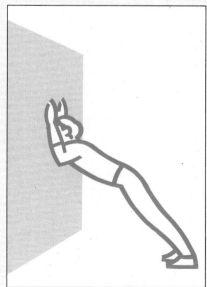

# Choosing
# an Exercise

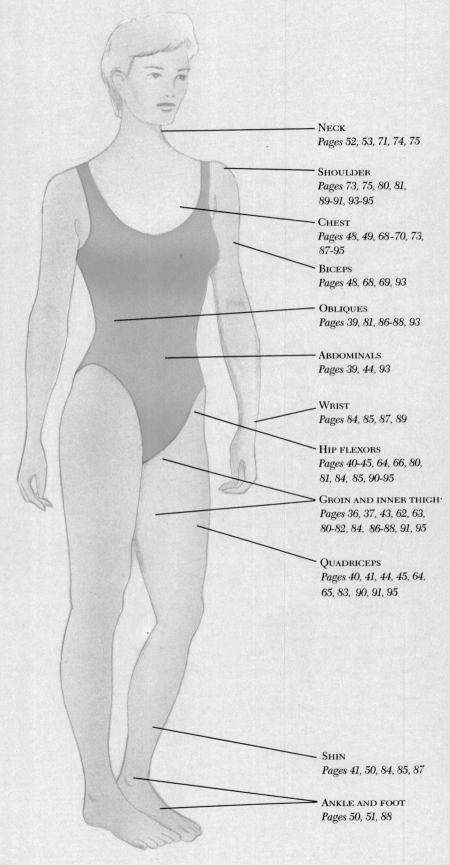

Once you have taken the flexibility tests on pages 18-19 and determined which of your muscles need improvement, you can use the illustrations at right to select the most appropriate exercises in this book. You do not have to perform every exercise listed for each muscle group; one or two will usually be enough. But you can try each exercise to find the ones you are most comfortable with.

If you engage in another form of exercise or play sports and you wish to use stretching routines as part of your warm-up and cool-down, turn to Chapter Four. There you will find stretching routines for eight of the most popular recreational sports.

The dynamic movement routines in Chapter Five are stretches that work the body as a whole, rather than isolating specific muscles and muscle groups. Therefore, the illustrations here do not refer to those routines.

Whatever exercises you choose, be sure to read the following four pages in order to perform the exercises safely and effectively.

NECK
*Pages 52, 53, 71, 74, 75*

SHOULDER
*Pages 73, 75, 80, 81,
89-91, 93-95*

CHEST
*Pages 48, 49, 68-70, 73,
87-95*

BICEPS
*Pages 48, 68, 69, 93*

OBLIQUES
*Pages 39, 81, 86-88, 93*

ABDOMINALS
*Pages 39, 44, 93*

WRIST
*Pages 84, 85, 87, 89*

HIP FLEXORS
*Pages 40-45, 64, 66, 80,
81, 84, 85, 90-95*

GROIN AND INNER THIGH·
*Pages 36, 37, 43, 62, 63,
80-82, 84, 86-88, 91, 95*

QUADRICEPS
*Pages 40, 41, 44, 45, 64,
65, 83, 90, 91, 95*

SHIN
*Pages 41, 50, 84, 85, 87*

ANKLE AND FOOT
*Pages 50, 51, 88*

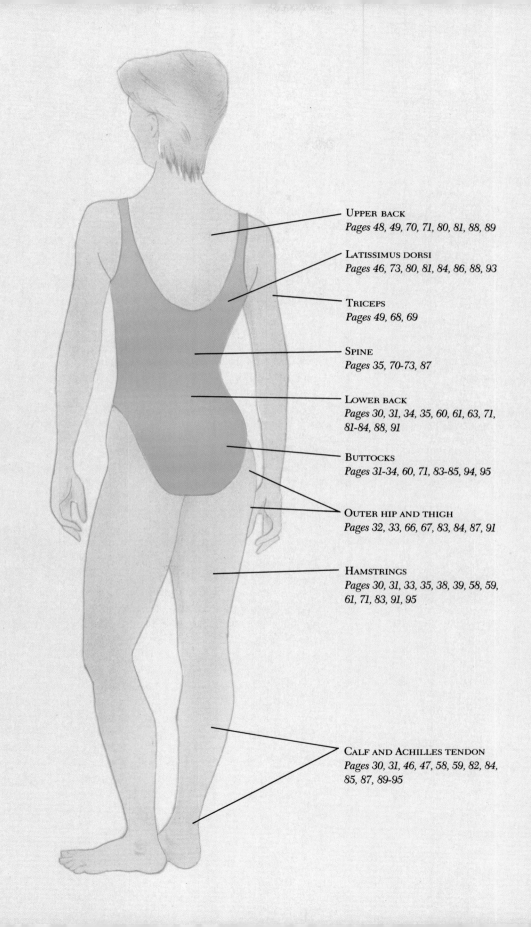

**UPPER BACK**
*Pages 48, 49, 70, 71, 80, 81, 88, 89*

**LATISSIMUS DORSI**
*Pages 46, 73, 80, 81, 84, 86, 88, 93*

**TRICEPS**
*Pages 49, 68, 69*

**SPINE**
*Pages 35, 70-73, 87*

**LOWER BACK**
*Pages 30, 31, 34, 35, 60, 61, 63, 71,
81-84, 88, 91*

**BUTTOCKS**
*Pages 31-34, 60, 71, 83-85, 94, 95*

**OUTER HIP AND THIGH**
*Pages 32, 33, 66, 67, 83, 84, 87, 91*

**HAMSTRINGS**
*Pages 30, 31, 33, 35, 38, 39, 58, 59,
61, 71, 83, 91, 95*

**CALF AND ACHILLES TENDON**
*Pages 30, 31, 46, 47, 58, 59, 82, 84,
85, 87, 89-95*

# Common Mistakes

## Relax When You Stretch

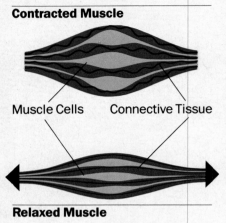

**Contracted Muscle**

Muscle Cells   Connective Tissue

**Relaxed Muscle**

When you try to stretch a contracted muscle *(top)*, as in performing ballistic stretches, proportionately more of the external force is placed on the muscle fiber than on the connective tissue. This may result in microscopic tears. When you stretch a relaxed muscle *(above)*, you stretch the connective tissue, which helps prevent injury.

A growing body of research suggests that some people who stretch to avoid injury when they work out or play sports can get injured from the stretches themselves. In one survey of 4,000 running injuries, stretching exercises were found to be a major cause of injury. The study also determined that those who were injured performed certain exercises that placed excessive stress on joints, ligaments and muscles. The most common of these are shown opposite. If you avoid these stressful stretches and observe the following precautions, you will be able to design a safe stretching program.

Perform slow static stretches, not bouncing or ballistic stretches such as leg kicks. Although studies show that ballistic stretches are as effective as static stretches for increasing flexibility, there is a possibility you will rupture ligaments and cause microscopic tears in your muscles. One reason for this is that bouncing causes the muscle to contract at the same time you are forcing it to stretch. Also, ballistic stretches are not as deliberate as static stretches, and the uncontrolled momentum of your limb may overload a joint and force it to move beyond its natural range of motion, very likely damaging the connective tissue.

Stretch your muscles only about 10 percent beyond their normal length. When a muscle is stretched to this limit, you should feel a comfortable tightness in the center of the muscle. Do not stretch any farther; if you feel discomfort at the muscle's end attachments, you are stretching too far and subjecting the tendon to too much tension. Never stretch to the point of pain. And remember that improving your flexibility is progressive — it cannot be done in one session. Forcing your muscles to stretch beyond their capability will cause injury and also loss of elasticity.

Always work within a joint's natural range of motion. If you force a joint to move beyond its natural range of motion, you may rupture or overstretch the ligaments. This can occur with certain dangerous stretches that place most of your body weight on one particular joint. Both the "plow" and the "hurdler's stretch" shown opposite can place excessive stress on certain joints. Deep knee bends can overstretch ligaments in the knees. Also, the ballet barre stretch can place a great deal of force on the extended knee, possibly damaging the cartilage and ligaments. This stretch can also compress the sciatic nerve, causing pain to radiate down the back of the legs from the buttocks.

Stretch before and after a strenuous workout session. A single stretching session will significantly improve flexibility and joint range of motion for at least 90 minutes. Stretching beforehand may reduce your chance of injury and improve your athletic performance. However, some athletic activities may tighten your muscles or cause delayed soreness. By stretching afterward, you can regain flexibility and prevent soreness.

If you do happen to become injured from overstretching, treat the injury like any other stress injury. Reduce the intensity of your exercises and apply ice packs to the affected area. Ice will lessen the discomfort and reduce the swelling. Of course, if you experience severe pain or if the discomfort of an injury lasts for several days, consult a physician.

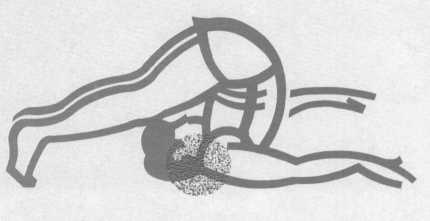

The plow *(left)* is a popular but dangerous stretch for the hamstring and back muscles. It places tremendous pressure on the back of the neck, which must support your entire body weight.

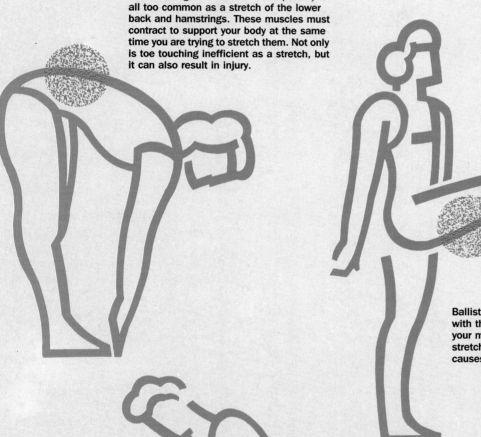

Toe touching with locked knees *(below)* is all too common as a stretch of the lower back and hamstrings. These muscles must contract to support your body at the same time you are trying to stretch them. Not only is toe touching inefficient as a stretch, but it can also result in injury.

Ballistic stretching, such as kicking your leg with the knee locked *(above)*, will stretch your muscles. But it will also induce the stretch reflex. This type of stretching often causes delayed localized muscle soreness.

The hurdler's stretch *(left)* should not be performed by anyone except very flexible athletes. The awkward twisting can cause strain and torn ligaments in the bent knee.

23

# The Training Regimen

Training your muscles to stretch farther is similar in concept to training them for strength: You must use the overload principle. Just as the only way to strengthen muscles is to exercise them slightly beyond their normal capacity and then progressively increase the workload, so to increase their flexibility you must follow a progressive stretching program.

As you advance in a flexibility program, you will not see steady improvement from one day to the next. Muscle soreness, motivation, ability to relax, room temperature and warm-up preparation are among the factors that influence your range of motion. But regardless of your flexibility at any particular time, by following the guidelines here, you should notice an improvement in a month.

### HOW HARD
Studies show that you should stretch a muscle about 10 percent beyond its normal length in order to increase its flexibility. At this point, you should be stretching about as far as you can without feeling pain. If you do feel pain, consider it a warning to ease up on the stretch.

### HOW OFTEN
You should stretch at least three days a week in order to obtain minimum benefits. For optimal results, however, you should stretch four to seven days a week.

### HOW LONG
Most experts agree that you should hold a stretch between 10 and 60 seconds to effectively lengthen a muscle. For the best results, however, you should stretch a muscle or muscle group for 15 to 30 seconds, pause and then repeat the stretch once or twice.

# Special Situations

If you spend long periods sitting or standing, or if you are so busy during the day that you do not have time for a full workout, you can benefit from the following exercises.

### SITTING
When you sit a lot, tension builds up in your lower back, shoulders and neck. Sitting for extended periods of time can also shorten your hamstrings and hip flexors and cause soreness in your buttocks. This set of exercises will counteract tension and discomfort in these areas. Half of them can be done while you are sitting.
• Hamstring stretch on a stool, page 31.
• Buttocks, pages 32-33.
• Hip-flexor stretch on a stool, page 43.
• Seated back stretch, page 35.
• Seated chest, back and shoulder stretches, page 49.
• Neck stretches, pages 52-53.

### STANDING
The strain of prolonged standing is usually felt in the muscles of your feet, calves, hips and lower back. These exercises are performed standing upright, and you can do them anytime, anywhere.
• Foot and shin stretches, pages 50-51.
• Calf stretches, page 47.
• Hamstring stretch on a stool, page 31.
• Hip-flexor stretch, page 42.
• Chest stretch against a wall, page 48.
• Full-body circle for the sides, shoulders, hips and back, pages 116-117.

### QUICK STRETCHING
If your time is limited, doing only a few stretches is better than doing none or trying to hurry through a full routine. Here is a round-up of stretches that you can complete in five minutes.

• Calf stretches, page 47.
• Hamstring stretch on a stool, page 31.
• Hip-flexor stretch against a wall, page 43.
• Roll down for back, hips and neck, pages 100-101.
• Full-body circle, pages 116-117.
• Diagonal reach for the shoulders, sides and inner thigh, pages 110-111.

# Ten Guidelines for Stretching

**1. CHOOSE THE BEST TIME OF DAY.**

Find a period when you are not likely to be interrupted by phone calls or other distractions. Proper stretching requires concentration and patience. Be sure that you do not rush through your routines. Also, do not work out immediately after a meal; a full feeling will make you uncomfortable.

**2. WEAR LOOSE-FITTING CLOTHING.**

Special exercise outfits are not essential for a stretching program, but you should wear loose, comfortable clothing that does not restrict your movement. To achieve the best results, you should stretch on a carpeted floor in bare feet. For comfort's sake, do not wear a belt or jewelry.

**3. WARM UP.**

Perform a five- to 10-minute aerobic warm-up, such as jogging in place or stationary cycling, before you stretch. You will be adequately warmed up when you begin to sweat. Warming up helps increase the circulation and temperature in your muscles, which in turn increases their pliability. Stretching muscles that are cold is less effective than stretching them when they are warmed up.

**4. LISTEN TO YOUR BODY.**

Remember that your flexibility changes from day to day and you may not be able to perform the same stretch on one day that you did the day before. Never try to force a stretch; instead, ease into it and take the muscle only to the point of slight discomfort. The stretch should always occur in the center of the muscle, not at the attachments, and should never cause pain.

**5. BREATHE EVENLY.**

The key to stretching is to remain relaxed during your exercises. Breathing rapidly or irregularly or holding your breath may make you tense. Instead, go into a stretch as you are exhaling, then concentrate on breathing normally and slowly.

**6. BE SPECIFIC.**

Flexibility does not diffuse itself throughout the body. Achieving flexibility in part of the body, or having stretched a particular muscle, does not mean that you will necessarily gain flexibility in another area. Be sure to pay special attention to those body areas that are the least flexible and stretch them more often.

**7. DO STRETCHES IN PAIRS.**

Work for bilateral flexibility — that is, equal flexibility on both sides of your body. When stretching one side of the body, be sure to follow with the same stretches on the other side.

**8. PROGRESS AT YOUR OWN SPEED.**

Do not attempt to force your muscles into flexibility. Begin slowly and gradually work toward your goals. Never try to compete with another person by seeing who can stretch farther. Flexibility is an individual matter.

**9. TAKE EXTRA TIME IF NECESSARY.**

If you have been inactive for a while and your muscles are unaccustomed to being stretched, then you should start slowly. The same is true if you have muscle soreness as the result of a stress injury from overdoing a sport or exercise. However, never stretch muscles that are torn or strained; you will only worsen the condition.

**10. KEEP TRACK OF YOUR PROGRESS.**

Test your general flexibility (*pages 18-19*) at the beginning of your training program to establish your flexibility baseline. Then retest your suppleness monthly as you progress. Once you have achieved the flexibility you want, continue stretching about three times a week to maintain your level.

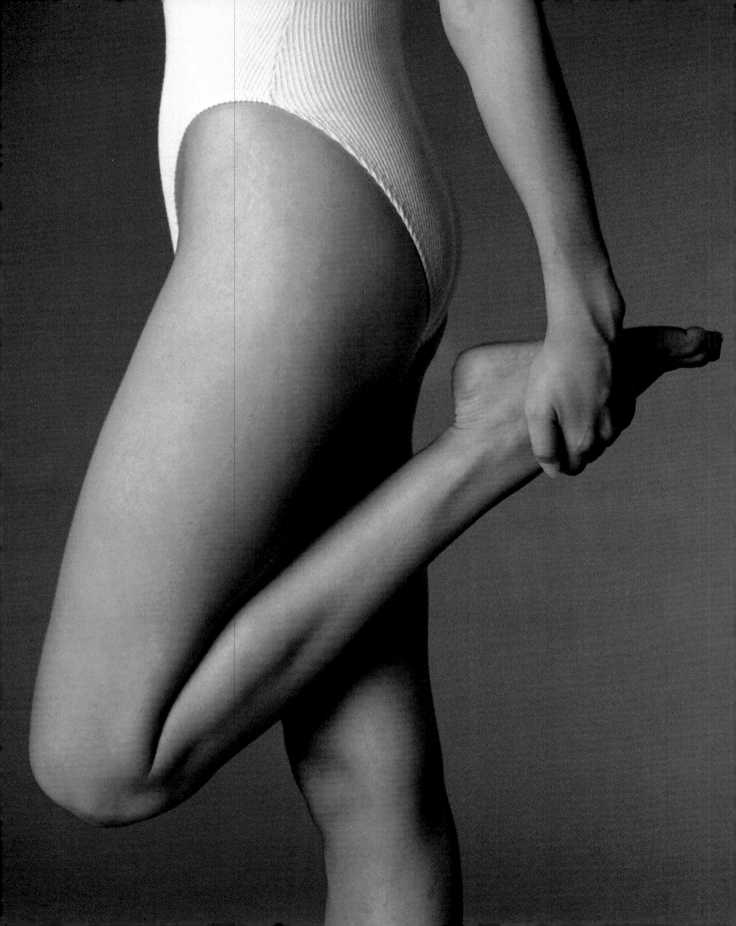

# CHAPTER TWO

# Basic Stretching

*A whole-body routine for greater
flexibility and better posture —
anytime, anywhere*

Static stretching, also known as
sustained or passive stretching, is by far the most popular technique
for improving flexibility. It is safe, convenient and pain-free. You can
perform static stretches whenever and wherever you want. You can do
them standing up, sitting or lying down. And you do not need a coach,
a trainer, exotic exercise equipment or a health club. All that is required for most static stretches is loose, comfortable clothing, a wall or
another solid surface to lean against and, occasionally, a chair or bench
to support you.

One of the great advantages of static stretching is that it helps you
become better acquainted with the interrelationships of your body's
muscles and tendons. Its slow, deliberate movement teaches you to
feel how your muscles work in groups. You will become more aware of
muscle tension, contraction and relaxation; and you will be able to
isolate particular muscle groups to determine which are tighter or less
flexible than others. By recognizing the limits of your muscles' flexibili-

ty, you can avoid overstretching and injury; furthermore, you will be better able to gauge the improvement in your flexibility.

Static stretching involves a slow pull that extends a muscle just beyond its normal length. Continued pressure holds the muscle in a stretched position for a sustained period. To benefit from static stretching, you must hold the stretch for at least six seconds. However, to get the best results, you should hold a stretch from 15 to 30 seconds and then repeat the exercise once or twice. The stretching must be forceful enough to enhance flexibility but not so rigorous as to cause injury to the muscles or tendons. Most experts agree that you should perform static stretches to the point of mild discomfort but never stretch so far that you feel acute pain. While stretching can help alleviate muscle soreness, it can also cause soreness when overdone. If you are just starting a stretching program, therefore, you should be especially careful that you do not overstretch a muscle.

Because a static stretch is gentle and prolonged, the technique reduces the muscle-spindle stretch reflex, which would normally cause the muscle to contract when it is stretched *(see box page 10)*. For this reason, mild static stretches are superior to forceful ballistic stretches, in which a person bounces or swings part of his or her body to gain momentum and force a stretch. Ballistic stretching causes the muscle spindles to induce a reflexive contraction in the very muscle you are trying to stretch. As long as your stretch is slow and deliberate, however, you can safely lengthen a muscle beyond its normal reach as you develop flexibility.

Static stretching is most effective when you can apply an external force to aid your stretch. As the stretching exercises on the following pages show, there are a number of ways to do this. For example, you can induce a static stretch of your chest muscle simply by drawing your arm as far back as possible and holding it there. But that stretch is limited by the flexibility of your chest muscle and by the strength of the opposing muscles on the other side of the shoulder joint pulling your arm back. The weaker those muscles, the less effective the stretch. You can get a much better stretch of the chest muscle by bracing your hand against a wall and twisting your body away from the wall. Then you do not have to rely on the strength of your chest's opposing muscles; instead, your leg and trunk muscles are able to apply greater force by using the wall for leverage. You will be able to hold the stretch for a longer time without the opposing muscle becoming fatigued.

Another way to introduce an external force to enhance static stretching is to apply the leverage of one or more limbs against that of another. You can, for instance, support yourself against a wall or lie face down on the ground and grasp your ankle, pulling it toward your buttocks. This technique will stretch your quadriceps on the front of your thigh far more effectively than if you tried to stretch them by contracting your opposing hamstring muscles and lifting your foot without external assistance.

## Getting Started: The Elongation Stretch

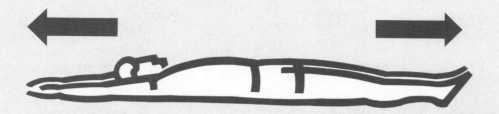

A simple and easy stretch that will help you release muscular tension is the elongation stretch, shown above. You should precede every stretching session with this exercise. Lie face up on the floor, stretching your arms out and bringing your legs together. Extend your arms and legs as far as you can, pointing your fingers and toes out, your palms facing the ceiling. Tilt your pelvis toward the floor so that you gently extend the curve of your back. Tuck your chin in. Hold this stretch for about 10 seconds, then relax. Repeat three times.

The elongation stretch is a full-body routine: You should feel the stretch in the top of your feet, your ankles, shins, abdominals, chest, sides, shoulders, lower back, upper back and arms. When performing the elongation stretch, be sure to breathe deeply and slowly. Shallow or rapid breathing can cause muscular tension.

Gravity, too, can play a role in stretching. When you lean into a wall with one or both legs extended backward, gravity pulls your body down and applies force to the musculature of your lower leg, thereby stretching your calf muscles.

When you embark on a static stretching program, give yourself plenty of time to stretch. Do not hurry through it. Be sure you are properly supported so that you do not lose your balance. Too often, for instance, people try to perform a quadriceps stretch by pulling their heel back to their buttocks while trying to balance on one foot. Stretching in this manner not only causes undue muscular tension in the supporting leg, but the unsteady stance can diminish the effectiveness of the stretch.

At the beginning of your stretching program, you may notice inappropriate contractions, chiefly in the opposing muscles. For instance, while stretching your hamstrings you might feel a tense quivering or tightening of the quadriceps. These muscle contractions are normal. Some people embarking on a stretching program also report a temporary numbness in some muscles while they stretch them. As you gain experience and develop better flexibility and control, both the contractions and sensations of numbness should disappear; your muscles should feel a warm tightness as they are being stretched and a pleasant looseness afterward.

# Hamstrings

A group of three large muscles in the back of the thigh, the hamstrings are among your body's most important muscles, since they act to straighten the hip and bend and rotate the knee. Virtually every sport and physical activity makes use of these muscles, and, as a result, they are frequently subject to tightness and stress injuries.

In the stretching routines that follow, many of the exercises are shown for only one side of the body: For example, in the hamstring stretch at right, the left leg is being stretched. When you do this or any other exercise that stretches muscles on either the right or the left, be sure to repeat the exercise for the other side of the body.

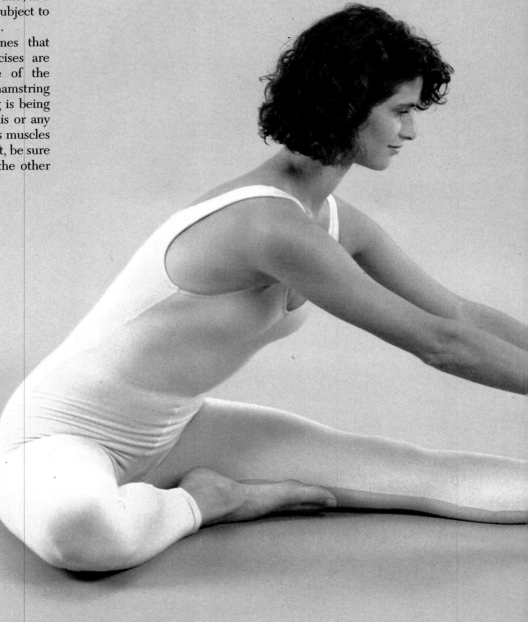

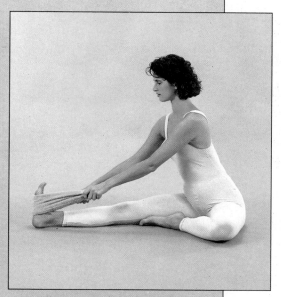

Sit on the floor with one leg extended and the other leg bent at the knee. Loop a towel around your foot and pull your leg. This is a good stretch if you have particularly tight hamstrings and calves.

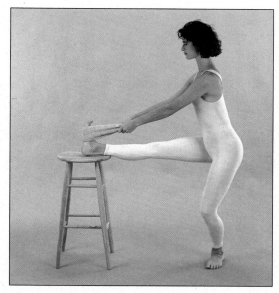

Place your heel on a stool and loop a towel around your foot. With your standing knee bent, pull your leg into the stretch. Be sure to keep your back straight.

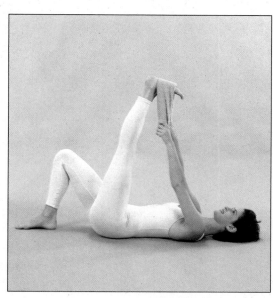

Lie on your back with one foot on the floor and the other leg extended in the air. Loop a towel around the foot of your extended leg and draw it toward you as far as you can.

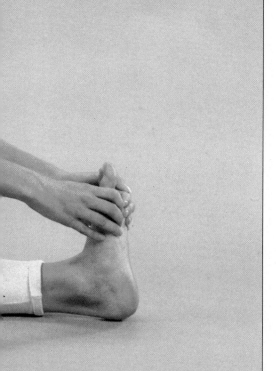

Sit on the floor with one leg extended and the opposite knee bent. Keeping your back straight, lean forward slowly to grasp your toes. This will stretch your hamstrings, lower back and calf muscles.

# Buttocks

The buttocks region is composed of nine major muscles. They include the gluteals, which straighten the hip, rotate the thigh and take part in straightening the knee. Because the buttocks muscles stabilize the pelvis, they are particularly active while you walk. They can become strained with overuse, and they can tighten with inactivity. To prevent inflexibility in the buttocks muscles, you should perform at least one of the exercises on these two pages regularly.

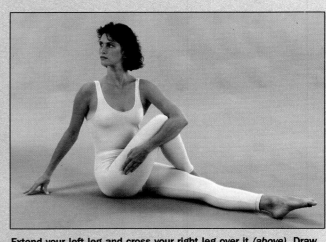

Extend your left leg and cross your right leg over it *(above)*. Draw your right knee back with your left arm. For a greater stretch, tuck your left foot under your right thigh *(below)*.

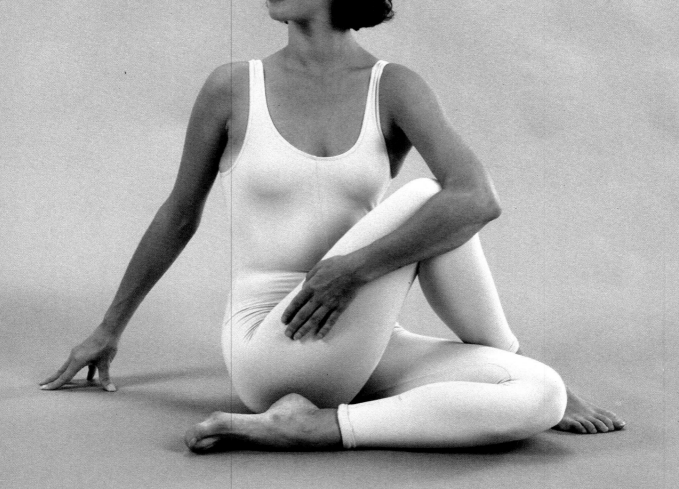

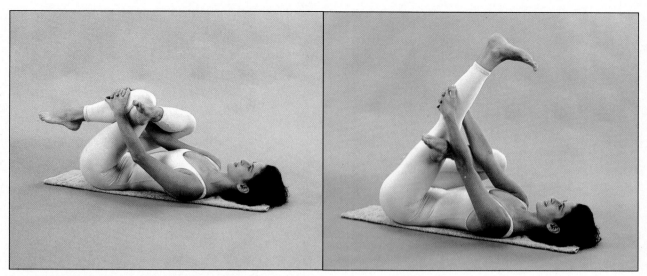

Stretch the muscles in your right buttocks by lying face up on the floor, resting your right ankle just above your left knee and drawing your knee toward your chest by pulling with both hands *(above)*. Then stretch the hamstrings as well as the buttocks by extending your left leg *(above right)*.

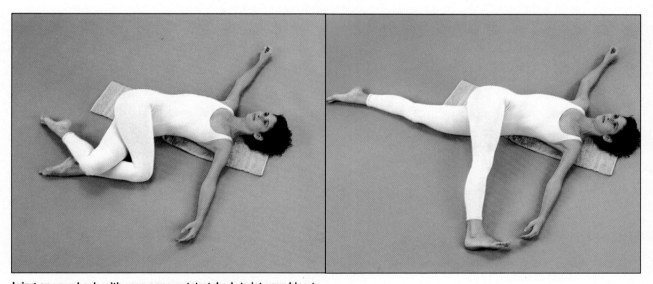

Lying on your back with your arms outstretched, twist your hips to the left and tuck your right calf under your left knee *(above)*. The weight of your left leg will help stretch the right buttocks muscles. For a hamstring stretch *(above right)*, straighten your left leg and extend the right leg; try to bring your toes to your left hand.

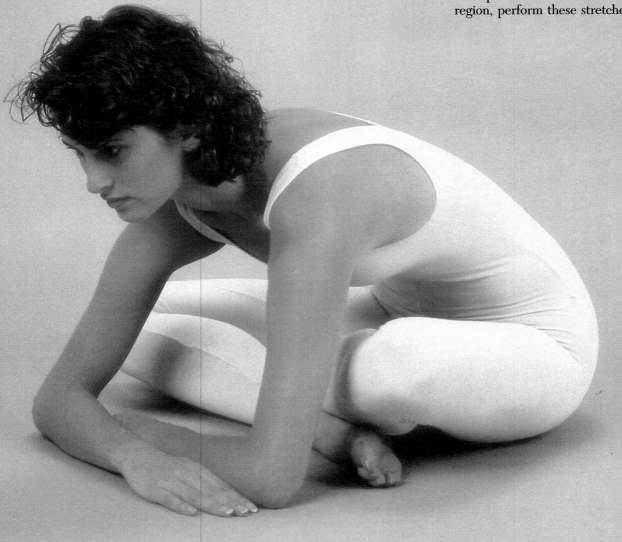

Sit on the floor with your legs crossed, then twist to the right and lean forward on your hands, stretching the lower back *(above)*. To stretch the lower back and buttocks, lean forward and bring your forearms toward the floor *(below)*.

# Lower Back

The muscles and connective tissues of the lower back support your upper body. Like the rigging on a ship's mast, the deepest layers of muscles anchored in the lower back rope up the entire spine and attach to the vertebrae. The latissimus dorsi — the muscle you use when you pull your elbow back — also attaches to the lower back region. No wonder, then, that the lower back is frequently the site of muscle and connective-tissue stress. Poor posture, of course, can exacerbate lower back pain. To relieve pain and reduce stress to the region, perform these stretches.

Sit on a stool or a chair with a high seat. Gently drop your body toward your lap, letting your hands dangle to the floor and your head drop between your legs.

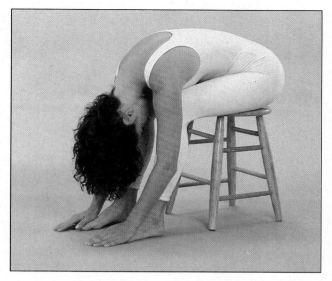

Lie on the floor, bend your knees and bring your feet toward your head. Hold on to your feet and pull your knees toward your chest to stretch your lower back and hamstrings.

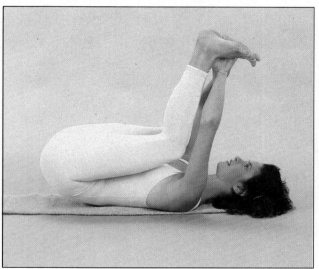

Kneel down and place your hands on the floor with your elbows extended and your back straight. Curl up like a cat by arching your back.

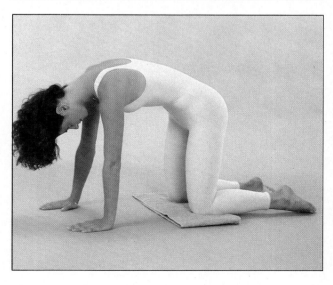

# Inner Thighs/1

The muscles of the inner thigh and groin area are called the adductors, since they adduct the thigh, or move it in toward the opposing leg. The adductors are connected to the lower portion of the pubic bone and run down the inside of the thighbone, where they attach along a tendinous strip. Many people who exercise regularly ignore their inner thigh muscles, allowing them to become short and tight. These muscles can then be easily injured, resulting in what are commonly called groin pulls. To reduce the chance of injury and to extend the range of motion in your legs, you should routinely stretch your inner thigh muscles with the exercises here and on pages 38-39.

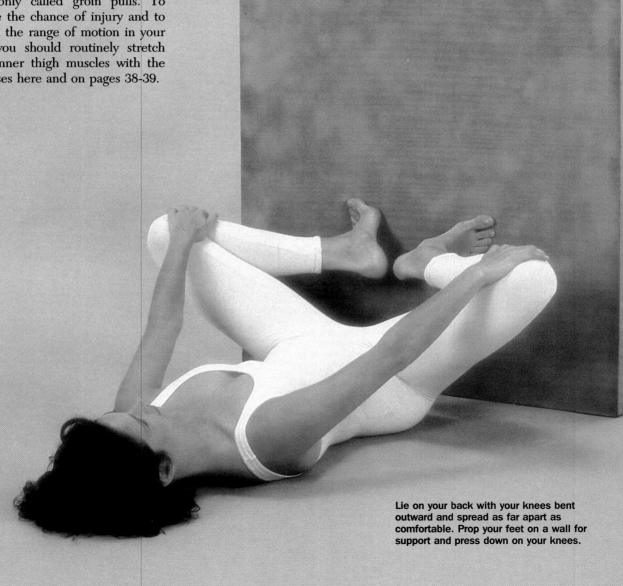

**Lie on your back with your knees bent outward and spread as far apart as comfortable. Prop your feet on a wall for support and press down on your knees.**

While lying on your back, extend your feet in the air and spread your legs as far apart as you can. Press down on your inner thighs with your arms.

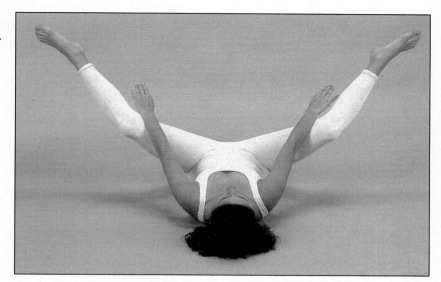

Draw one knee up and support it with your hand as you straighten your other leg, where you will feel a concentrated stretch.

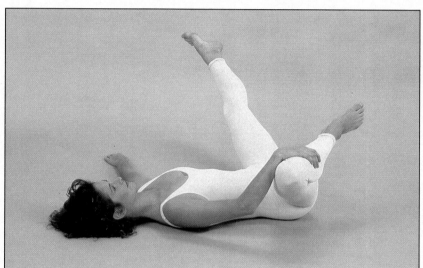

Bring the soles of your feet together and grasp your feet with your hands. Pull your feet toward you to stretch the inner thigh muscles closest to your groin area.

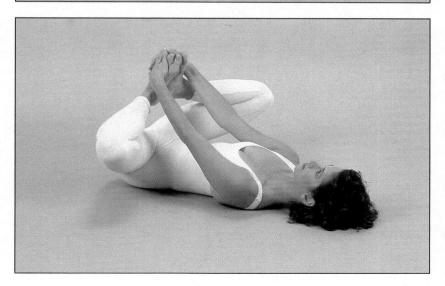

# Inner Thighs/2

With your legs stretched in front of you, straighten your knees and spread your legs as wide as you can. To stretch both the inner thigh muscles and the hamstrings, lean forward and rest on your elbows *(near right)*. To concentrate on the musculature in your right leg, rotate your torso to the right and reach toward your foot with your left hand *(far right)*. Then lean to the left and raise your right hand toward the ceiling to stretch the abdominals, obliques and other side muscles *(below)*.

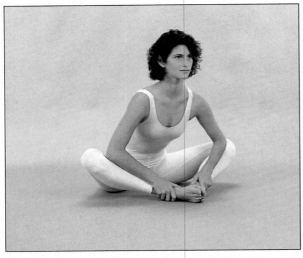

Sit on the floor with the soles of your feet together. Grasp your feet and lean forward, pressing your forearms on your shins.

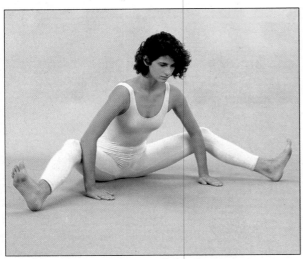

While still sitting, spread your legs as far apart as you comfortably can, keeping your knees bent. Lean forward from the waist and place your hands on the floor. Press against your knees with your elbows.

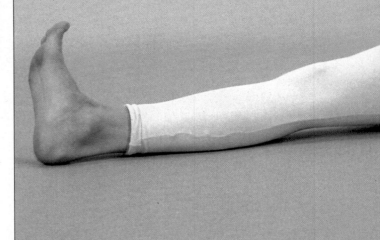

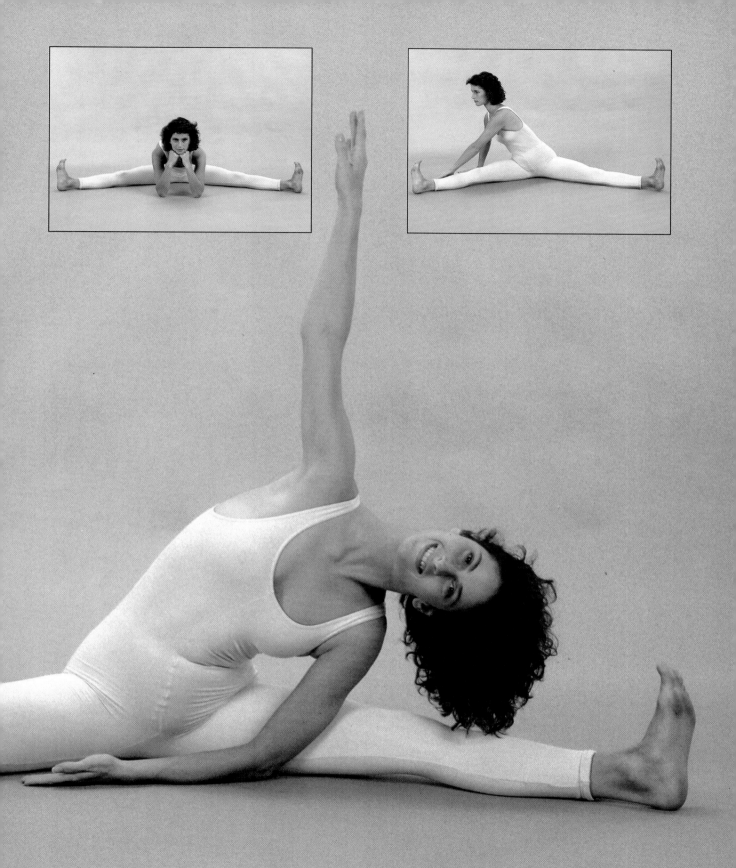

# Quadriceps and Hip Flexors/1

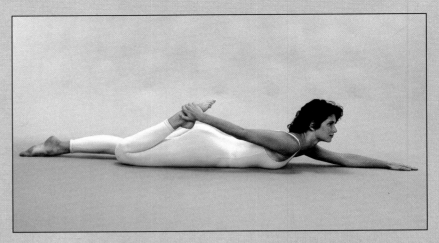

The quadriceps are four thigh muscles that begin on the hipbone and the thighbone and become united on a single tendon that is attached to the kneecap. These muscles work together primarily to straighten the knee. The hip flexors are a group of muscles, including one of the quadriceps, that lift your thigh. Tight quadriceps and hip flexors can limit your ability to run and jump. In addition, tight hip flexors can tilt your pelvis forward and lead to lordosis, or excessive curvature of the lower back.

**Lie on your stomach and grasp your right foot with your right hand. Pull your heel to your buttocks to stretch the quadriceps *(above)*. To stretch the hip flexors, pull your knee off the floor *(below)*.**

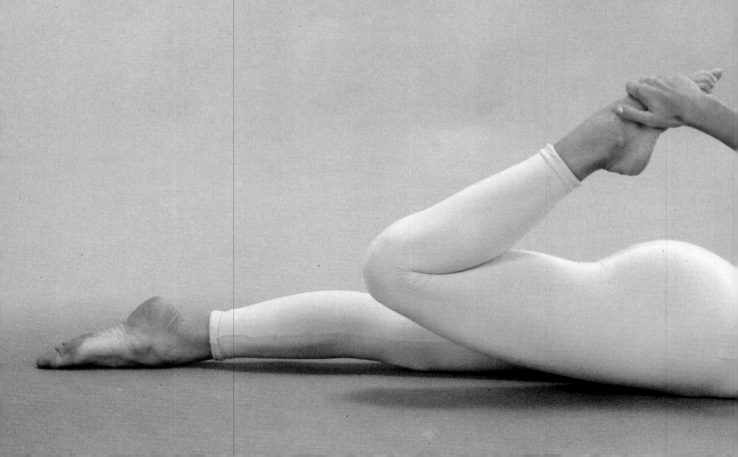

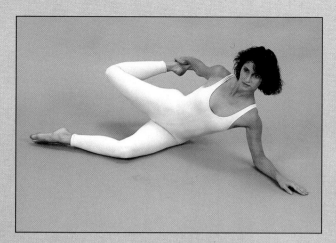

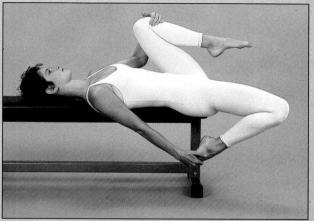

Lie on your left side and grasp your right foot with your right hand *(above left)*. Pull back on your foot until you feel a stretch of the quadriceps and hip flexors. Lie face up on an exercise table with your left leg tucked toward your chest, grasping the knee with your left hand *(above right)*. Extend your right leg over the edge of the table. Pull on your foot with your right hand. To stretch the hip flexors and shin muscles, stand facing away from a stool. Using a wall for balance, rest the top of your right foot on the seat *(right)*. Bend your left knee until you feel the stretch.

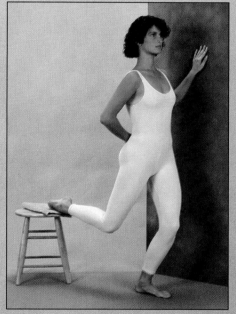

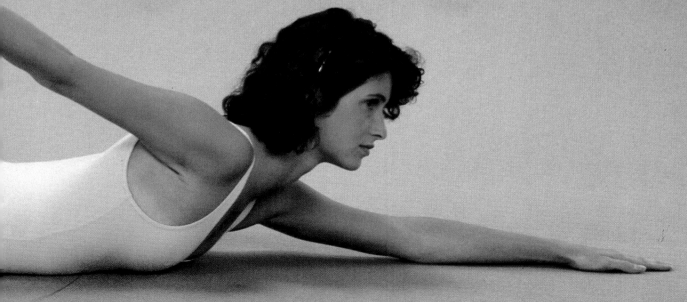

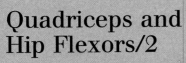

# Quadriceps and Hip Flexors/2

**Take an exaggerated step forward with your right foot. Brace yourself on your right knee and extend your left leg backward to stretch the hip flexors.**

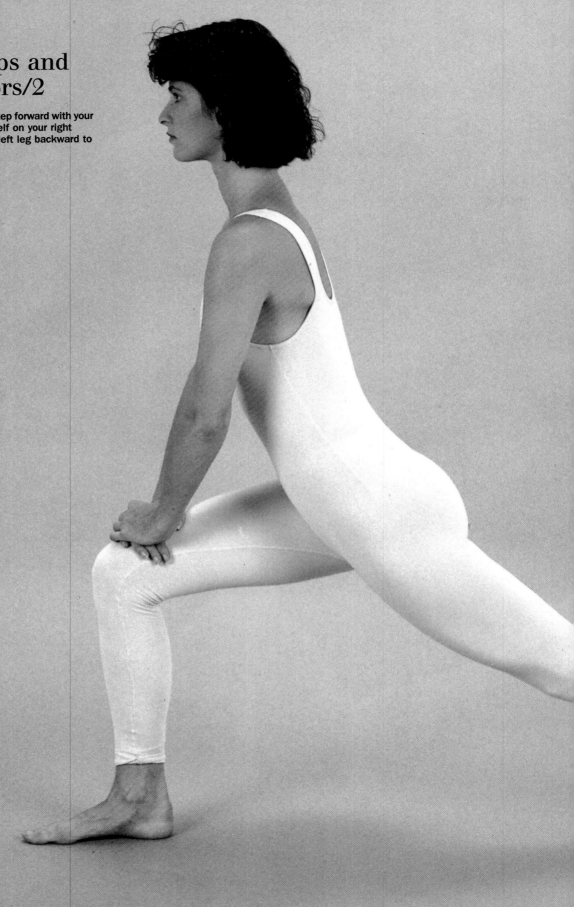

Kneel on your left leg with your right foot flat on the ground, turned out at the same angle as your right shoulder. To increase the stretch and include the right inner thigh, lean farther over your right foot.

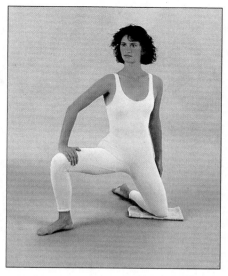

Perform a lunge stretch by using a wall for balance. Place your palms against the wall and extend your right leg behind you to stretch the hip flexors.

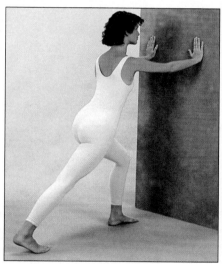

Place your right foot on the seat of a stool for a lunge variation. The higher the stool, the greater the stretch you can achieve. Grasp your shin and lean forward to lengthen the hip flexors in your left leg.

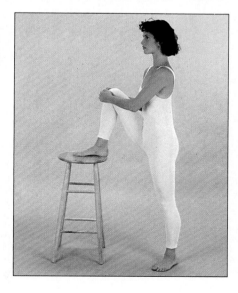

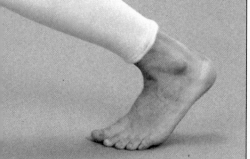

# Quadriceps and Hip Flexors/3

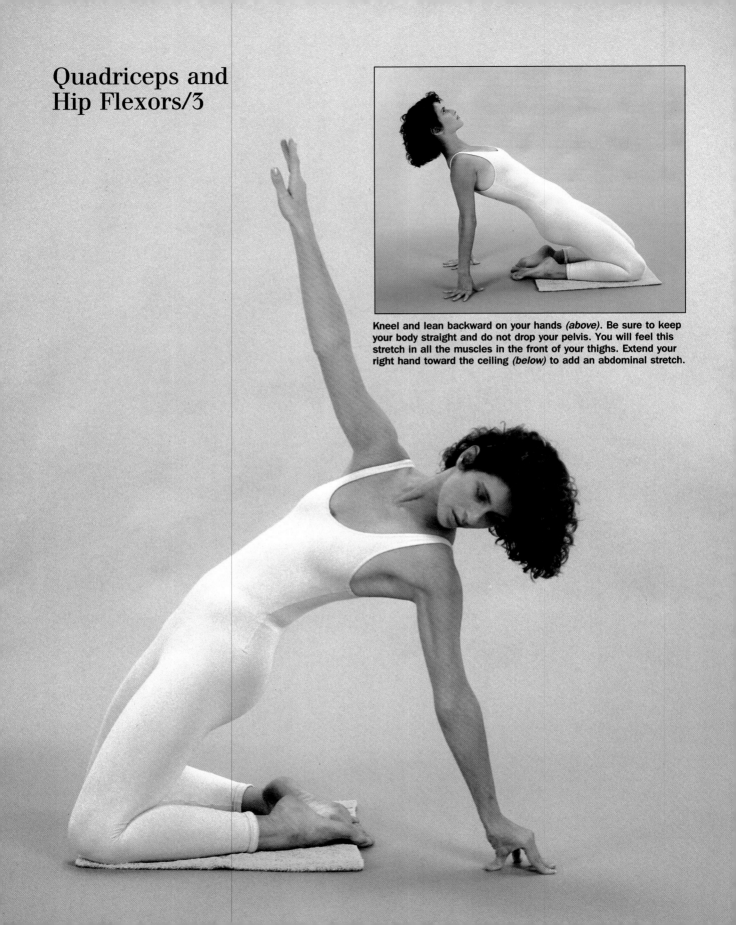

Kneel and lean backward on your hands *(above)*. Be sure to keep your body straight and do not drop your pelvis. You will feel this stretch in all the muscles in the front of your thighs. Extend your right hand toward the ceiling *(below)* to add an abdominal stretch.

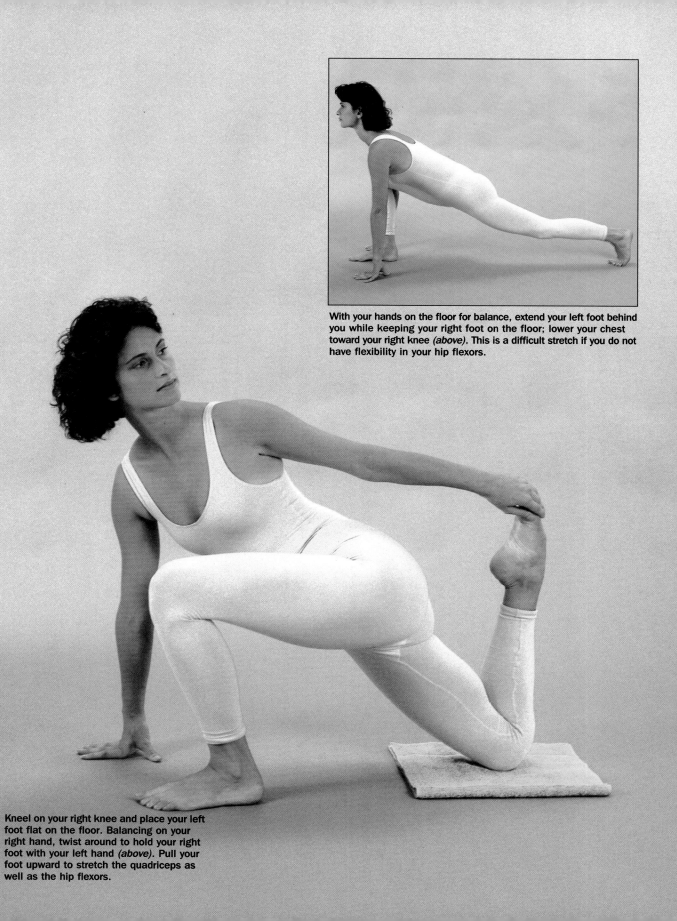

With your hands on the floor for balance, extend your left foot behind you while keeping your right foot on the floor; lower your chest toward your right knee *(above)*. This is a difficult stretch if you do not have flexibility in your hip flexors.

Kneel on your right knee and place your left foot flat on the floor. Balancing on your right hand, twist around to hold your right foot with your left hand *(above)*. Pull your foot upward to stretch the quadriceps as well as the hip flexors.

# Calves

Your calf muscle is composed of two distinct parts, the gastrocnemius and the soleus. The gastrocnemius is the large bulging muscle of the calf. It is connected to the Achilles tendon and is principally involved with lifting the heel off the ground and pushing off for walking, running and jumping. The soleus extends underneath the gastrocnemius and also connects to the Achilles tendon. Not as powerful as the gastrocnemius, the soleus pulls on the ankle joint when you stand on your toes.

Many people, especially those who run, have inflexible calf muscles. Tight calves can result in Achilles tendinitis, pronation, or inward roll of the foot, and plantar fascitis, an inflammation of the connective tissue in the sole of the foot.

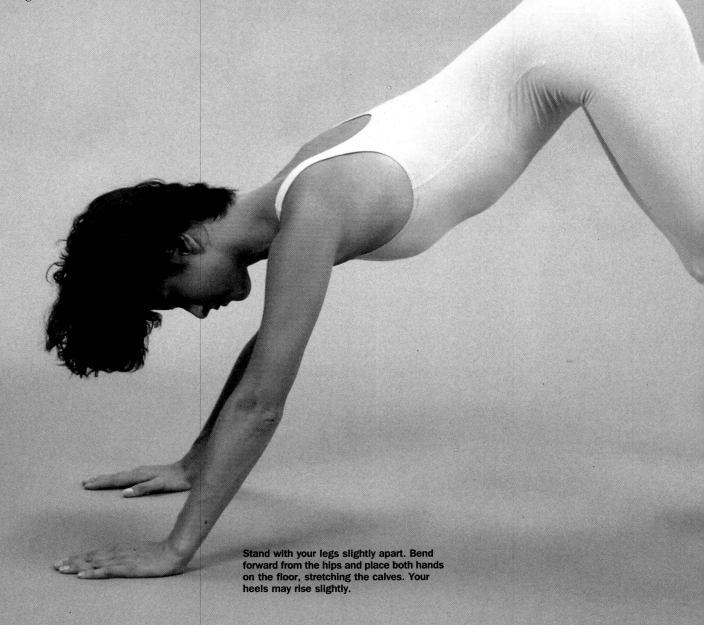

Stand with your legs slightly apart. Bend forward from the hips and place both hands on the floor, stretching the calves. Your heels may rise slightly.

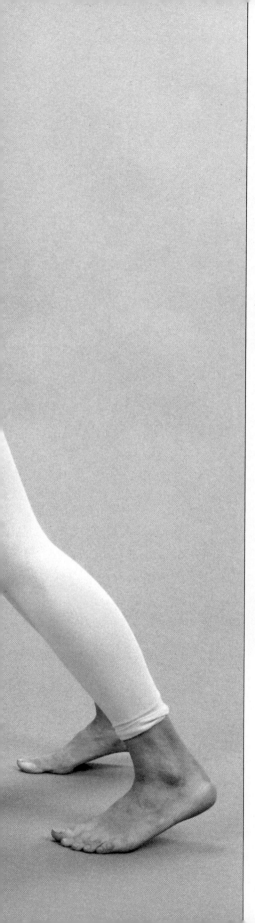

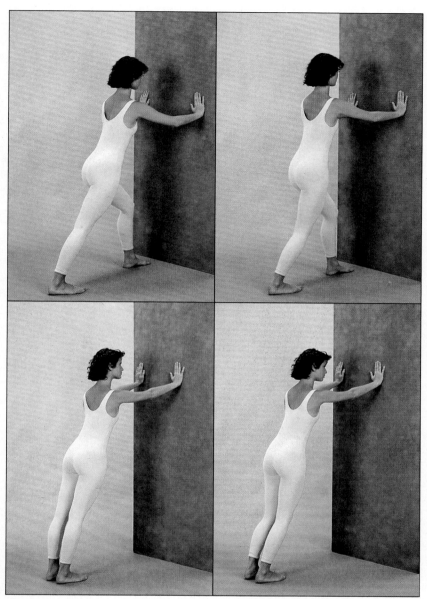

Place your palms against a wall, drawing your left knee forward and extending your right leg behind. Keep your right knee locked and your heel on the ground to stretch the gastrocnemius *(top left)*. To stretch the soleus, flex your right knee slightly *(top right)*. Lean into the wall with both feet extended behind you and both knees locked to stretch your left and right gastrocnemius muscles *(above left)*. Flex your knees slightly to include a soleus stretch in both legs *(above right)*.

# Upper Body

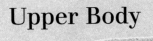

Stretching exercises for the upper body are important not only to protect you from muscle strain, but also to improve your posture and general appearance. Tight or weak chest and shoulder muscles, for instance, may result in rounded shoulders and bad posture, which are aggravated by sitting hunched over a desk all day. The upper body stretches on these two pages will help alleviate muscle tension in your chest and shoulders. You can perform the stretches on the opposite page while sitting at a desk.

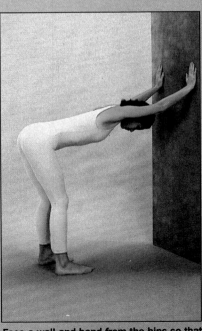

**Stand erect with your feet together. Grasp the ends of a towel with both hands and hold the towel behind your head** *(right)*. **This is a general stretch of the chest, shoulders and upper arms.**

**Face a wall and bend from the hips so that the top of your head points to the wall. Place your palms against the wall for a stretch of the shoulders and arms.**

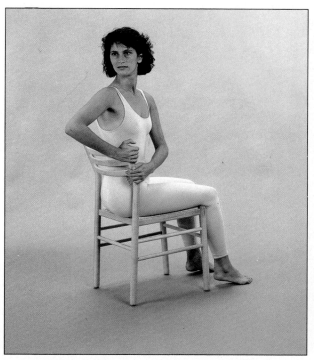

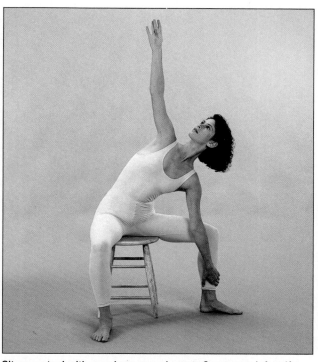

Sit upright in a straight-backed chair. Twist to the right and hold onto the chair frame. Pull back with your left arm and hold tight with your right to stretch your upper and middle back muscles.

Sit on a stool with your legs spread apart. Grasp your left calf with your left hand. Stretch your right hand toward the ceiling to elongate your chest and upper and middle back muscles.

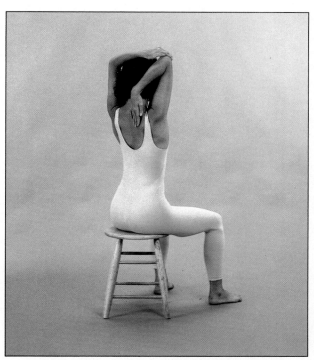

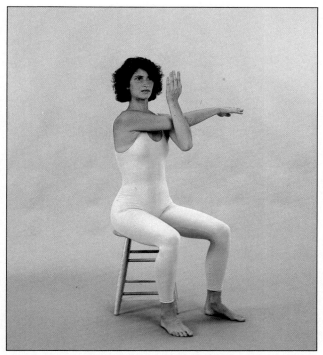

Sit upright with the palm of your right hand behind your neck. Grasp your right elbow with your left hand and pull it toward the back of your head, stretching the triceps of your right arm.

Sit on a stool and swing your right arm leftward across your chest. To enhance a stretch of the right triceps and shoulder, place your arm in the bend of your left elbow and pull up with your left arm.

# Feet

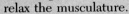

The foot is an amazingly complex structure that not only provides the strength to support your entire body, but also imposes subtle yet significant changes in pitch and direction to control your posture and gait. A well-functioning foot routinely absorbs tremendous force. Walking, for instance, subjects the foot to a force of up to 120 percent of your body weight with each step. Running subjects the foot to even greater loads — up to about five and a half times your body weight.

For all that the foot must do, it requires remarkably little care. Shoes that provide support and shock absorption are all that your feet normally need. In addition, stretching your feet helps increase circulation and relax the musculature.

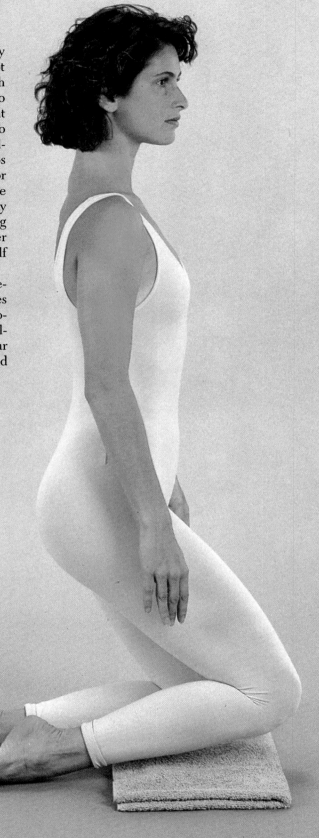

Sit comfortably in a chair with your foot off the floor and follow this sequence: First, extend your toes as far as you can, feeling the stretch from your ankle to your toes along the top of your foot *(right)*. Then turn your foot in *(far right)* to stretch the muscles along the outside of your foot. Pull your toes back toward your shin so that you feel tightness along the sole *(below left)*. Finally, turn out to lengthen the inside muscles *(below right)*.

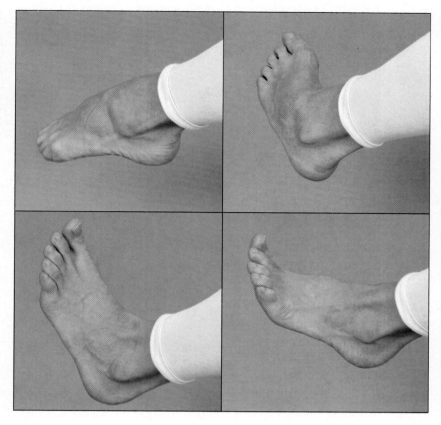

Kneel on the floor. Lift your right knee and draw it forward slightly *(opposite)*. Press the top of your right foot to the floor. This stretches the muscles of the metatarsal region, your ankle and shin.

# Neck

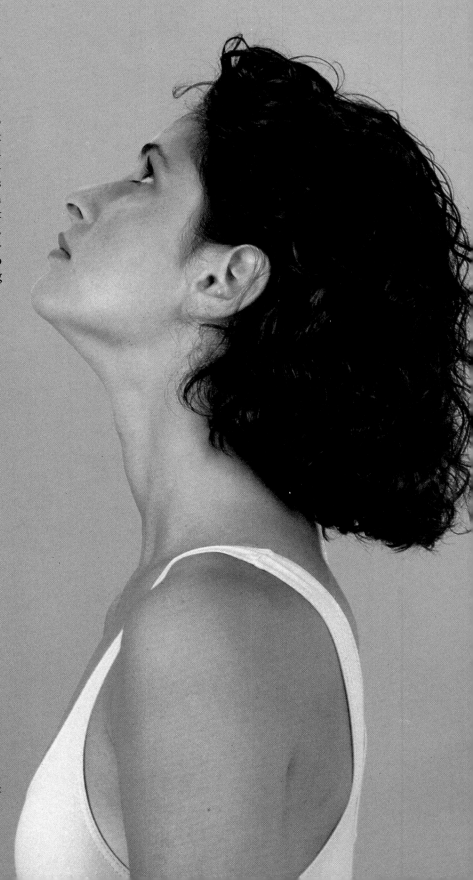

Not counting the larynx, your neck contains more than 30 muscles that act to rotate your head and to flex forward, backward and side to side. In addition to giving you this mobility, your neck must also protect your spinal cord and support your head. In daily living, these functions can sometimes be at odds, resulting in neck strain and stiffness. Regular exercise that requires extensive neck movements, such as cycling or swimming, can also cause neck strain. You can help prevent this problem by performing the exercises on these two pages.

**Drop your head backward to extend your neck. Do not force your neck back, but let your head drop naturally to lengthen the muscles along the front of your neck.**

Grasp the back of your head with your right hand, and pull it forward and to the right to stretch the trapezius.

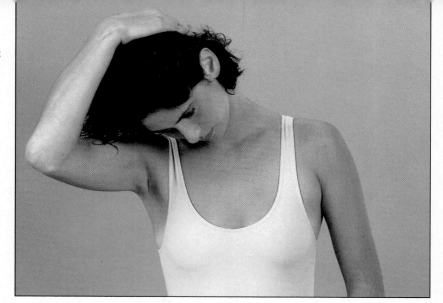

Place your right hand over your left ear, and pull your head to the right. This will stretch the mastoid muscle.

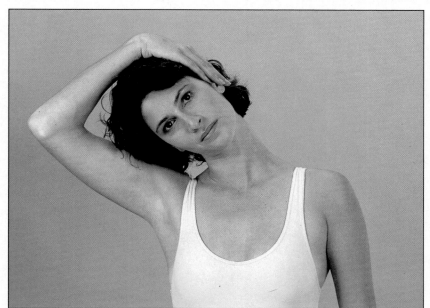

Interlace your fingers behind your head. Push your chin to your chest to lengthen the muscles in the back of your neck.

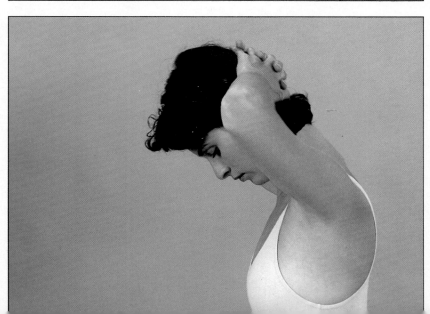

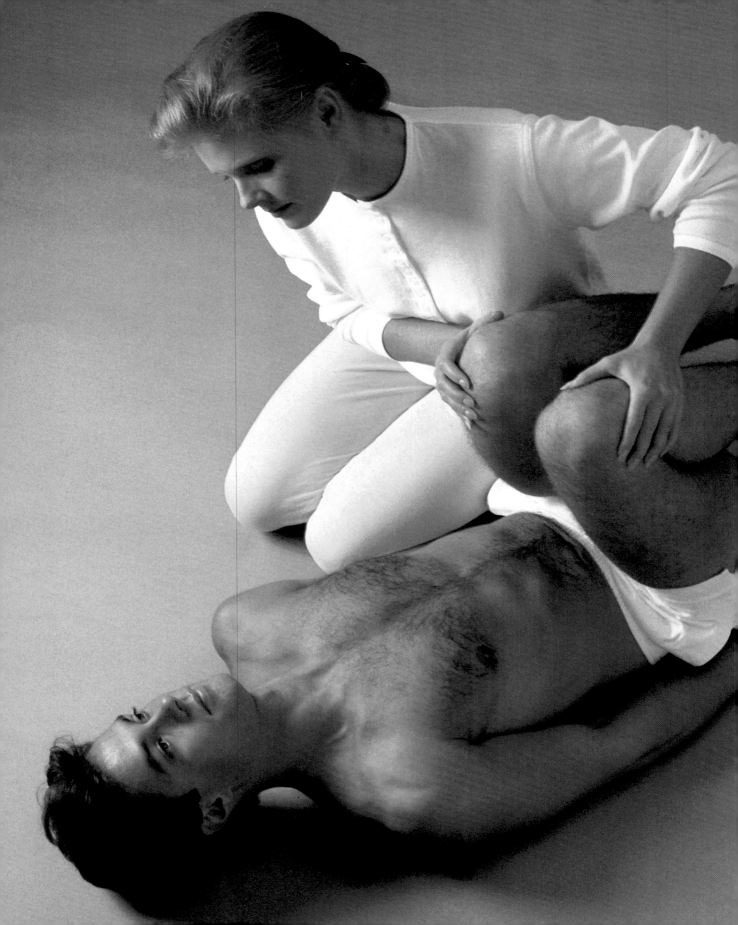

# CHAPTER THREE

# Partner Stretching

*Not only fun, but more effective*

P artner, or assisted, stretches involve two people: One person stretches and the other person helps to achieve the stretch. Assisted stretches can increase your range of motion farther than static, single-person stretches. The reason is simple: For most of the static stretches covered in Chapter Two, the muscle-stretching force is provided by body weight — applying the force of one limb on another or grasping an immovable object for leverage and then pulling. All these forces are limited by gravity or by your own strength. More effort and leverage can be applied to your limbs by a partner, increasing the length and duration of a stretch.

Partner stretching also allows you to perform a type of stretch called contract-relax. To carry out a contract-relax stretch, you must first perform a static stretch. Your partner holds the stretched limb in place while you push as hard as you can against the stretch with an isometric contraction. Then you release the contraction while your partner pushes your limb to a new point of tightness. You will find that this stretch is greater than what you can normally achieve. Although the contract-relax technique can sound complicated in theory, it is actually quite simple in practice *(see box opposite)*.

The contract-relax method of stretching has consistently proved more effective than traditional techniques. In one study, Swedish researchers asked two groups of subjects to stretch three times a week. One group used the ballistic method and the other the contract-relax technique. After 30 days, the researchers found that the contract-relax group had improved its flexibility more than twice as much as the ballistic-method group. The improvement in joint range of motion for those using the ballistic method averaged between 1.4 and 3.5 degrees, while improvement among those using the contract-relax technique averaged between 6.0 and 10.5 degrees.

In an American study comparing the contract-relax method with both ballistic and static stretching, subjects were randomly assigned to one of four groups: ballistic, static, contract-relax or control (no stretching at all). After a six-week, three-times-a-week flexibility-training program, the subjects were tested for flexibility of their shoulder, trunk and hamstring muscles. The results confirmed the Swedish tests, indicating that contract-relax techniques are superior to other stretching methods for improving flexibility.

Physiologists developed the contract-relax method as one of a group of therapies for paralyzed individuals. The doctors called this group of therapies proprioceptive neuromuscular facilitation, or PNF. Although a number of studies have documented the effectiveness of PNF techniques for lengthening muscles and increasing the range of motion, researchers do not agree on why this is so. The most widely accepted theory concerns the Golgi tendon organs, which are nerve fibers that sense tension in muscle tendons. During the contraction phase of the PNF routine, the tension caused by the strong pull of the isometric muscle contraction induces the Golgi tendon organs to send signals to the central nervous system. These signals, called inhibitory impulses, are part of a protective reflex response to prevent muscle and tendon tears. The inhibitory impulses override any signals from the muscle spindles to contract the muscle further. Then, when the muscle is stretching during the relax phase, the inhibitory impulses dampen the stretch-reflex response of the muscle spindles *(see box page 10)*. Although the neuromuscular process is complicated, the simple result is that you can stretch farther.

An added benefit of the contract-relax method is that it increases strength. According to one recent study, PNF stretching can be superior to weight training for improving athletic performance. Researchers randomly assigned 30 college women to one of three groups — a PNF group, a weight-training group and a control group. After training the women three times a week for eight weeks, the scientists found that the PNF group performed significantly better than either the weight-trained or the control group in both throwing and jumping abilities. Those women who trained with PNF exercises

## The Contract-Relax Method

To perform a contract-relax stretch, the basis for most of the routines in this chapter, your partner first guides you into a conventional static stretch. As you begin to feel the stretch, you reverse the motion and push against your partner as hard as you can. This is the contract phase, which is shown at top right for a stretch of the hamstring muscles. When you push against your partner, who provides immovable resistance, be sure to use only the muscles you are going to stretch. For example, in the hamstring stretch, you push with your thigh — which requires keeping your leg straight — not with your calf.

After five or six seconds, relax your muscles completely. Your partner then pushes the muscles back into a stretch that extends them farther than before. The two of you hold this position, shown at bottom right, for 20 to 30 seconds.

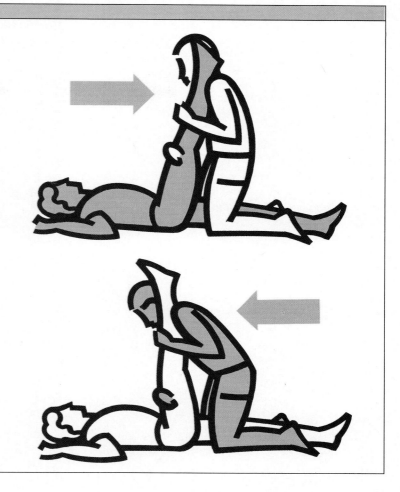

improved their throwing distance by 25 percent and their vertical-jump ability by 16 percent, while the weight-trained group had increases of only 12.8 and 9.9 percent, respectively. Many athletic coaches consider contract-relax routines an important component of their training programs.

Some contract-relax exercises can be performed without a partner. You can, for instance, stretch your inner thigh muscles by sitting cross-legged on the ground, pushing upward with your knees against the palms of your hands for the contract phase, then relaxing your inner thigh muscles and continuing to push down with your hands. But most PNF routines require another person to provide adequate isometric resistance during the first stretching phase and then strength to push you into the new stretch. The following pages offer a number of partner-assisted stretches, most of which involve the contract-relax method. Be sure to choose a partner who is sensitive to your needs and aware of your level of flexibility. He or she should stretch your muscles gently, until the stretch becomes slightly uncomfortable but not so far as to cause pain.

# Hamstrings and Calves

Your hamstrings, among the longest and strongest muscles in your body, are likely to become tight and inflexible if you do not stretch them regularly. This is also true of your calves, which form part of a biomechanical pulley system with the Achilles tendon, the heel and the plantar fascia along the bottom of the foot. The contract-relax method of stretching can be the most effective way to loosen the hamstrings and the calves. You can perform either the contract-relax stretch or a simple static stretch with your back on the ground, on a cushioned massage table or even on top of your kitchen table, putting a towel underneath you for comfort.

As in the previous chapter, any stretch that works muscles on one side of your body should be repeated for muscles on the other side.

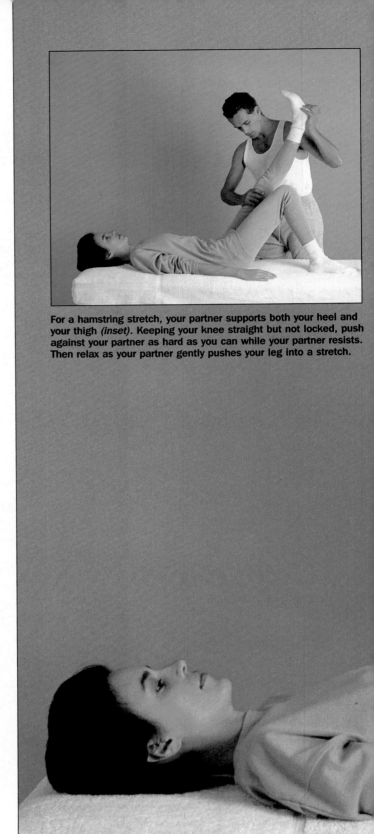

For a hamstring stretch, your partner supports both your heel and your thigh *(inset)*. Keeping your knee straight but not locked, push against your partner as hard as you can while your partner resists. Then relax as your partner gently pushes your leg into a stretch.

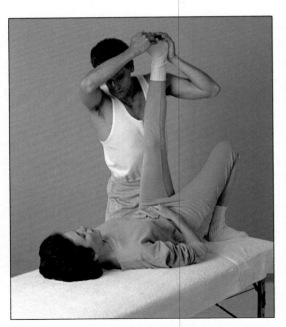

To perform a calf stretch, lie on your back with your knees flexed and your feet flat. Straighten one leg as your partner grasps your heel and draws it toward the ceiling. Push your leg against this stretching motion, then relax as your partner eases your leg into a new stretch.

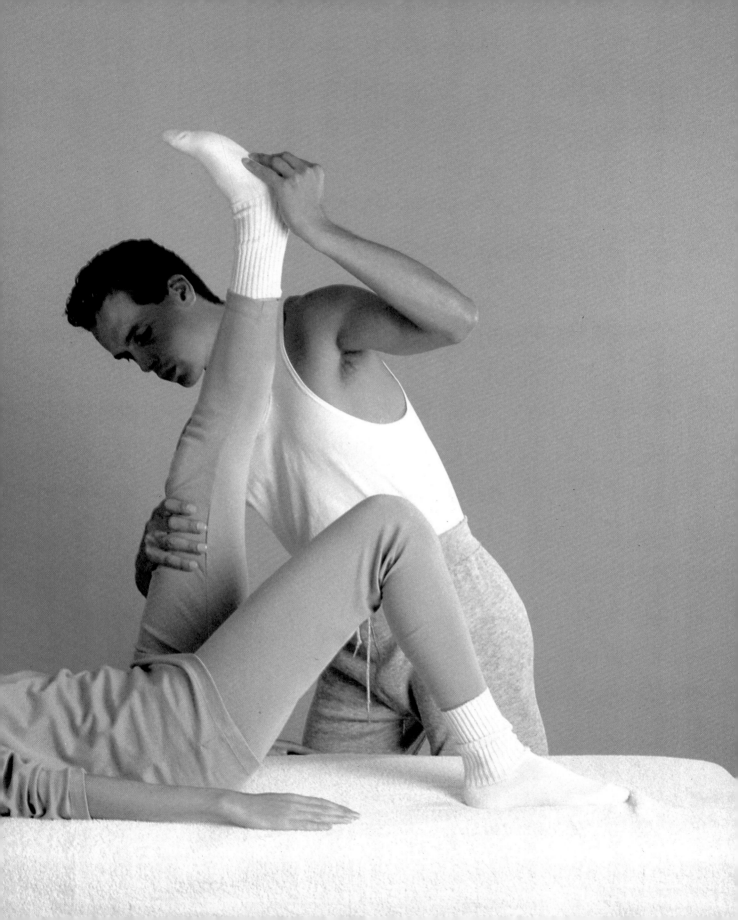

# Hamstrings and Lower Back

Since the hamstrings attach to the lower part of the pelvis, they frequently influence the lower back region. Tight hamstrings can tilt the pelvis and lead to an inflexible lower back. It makes sense, then, to stretch not only the hamstrings but also the lower back region. The partner-assisted stretches here will help ease tightness in your lower back as well as increase the flexibility of your hamstrings.

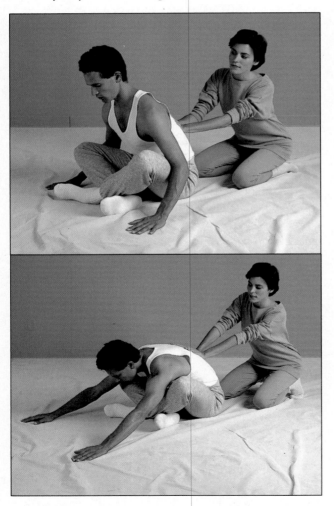

Sit cross-legged with your hands at your sides. Your partner kneels behind you and places her hands on your back *(top)*. Push against her, then reach forward to stretch *(above)*. This position stretches your lower back and some buttocks muscles.

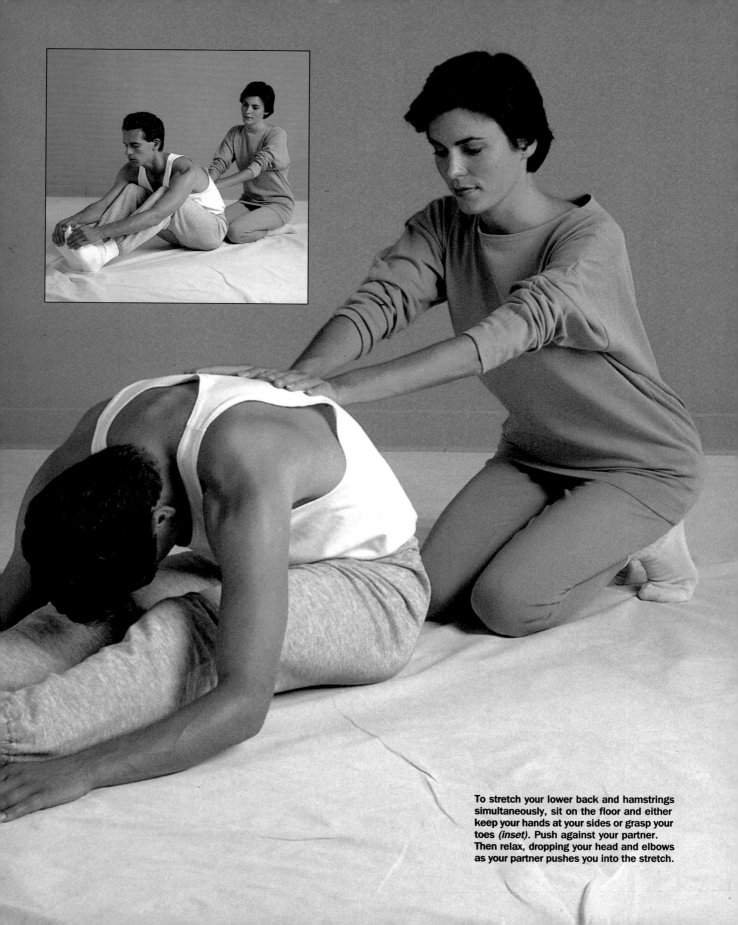

To stretch your lower back and hamstrings simultaneously, sit on the floor and either keep your hands at your sides or grasp your toes *(inset)*. Push against your partner. Then relax, dropping your head and elbows as your partner pushes you into the stretch.

# Inner Thighs

Many people — especially men — have tight inner thigh muscles, which can be particularly troublesome for those who are active. Recreational runners, for instance, frequently report pulled groin muscles. The inner thigh muscles, like the hamstrings and those of the lower back, are attached to the pelvis.

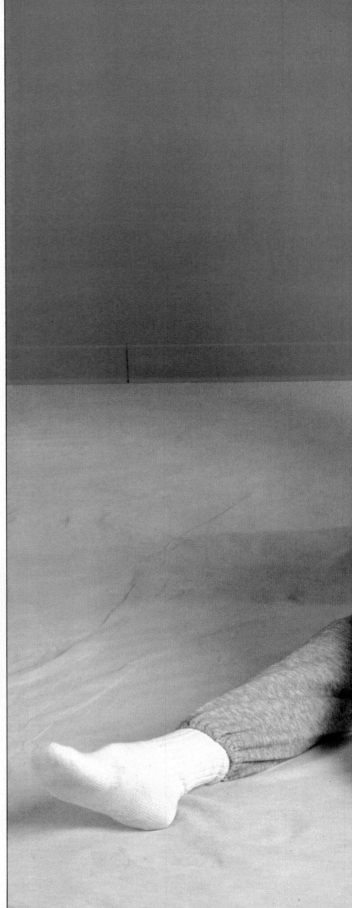

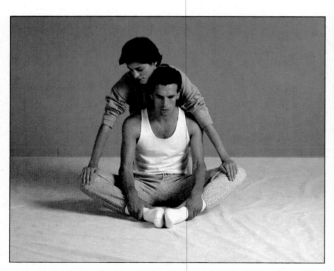

Sit cross-legged with the bottoms of your feet together. Your partner places her hands atop your knees while you attempt to push your knees upward. As you relax, your partner presses your knees toward the floor for the stretch *(above)*.

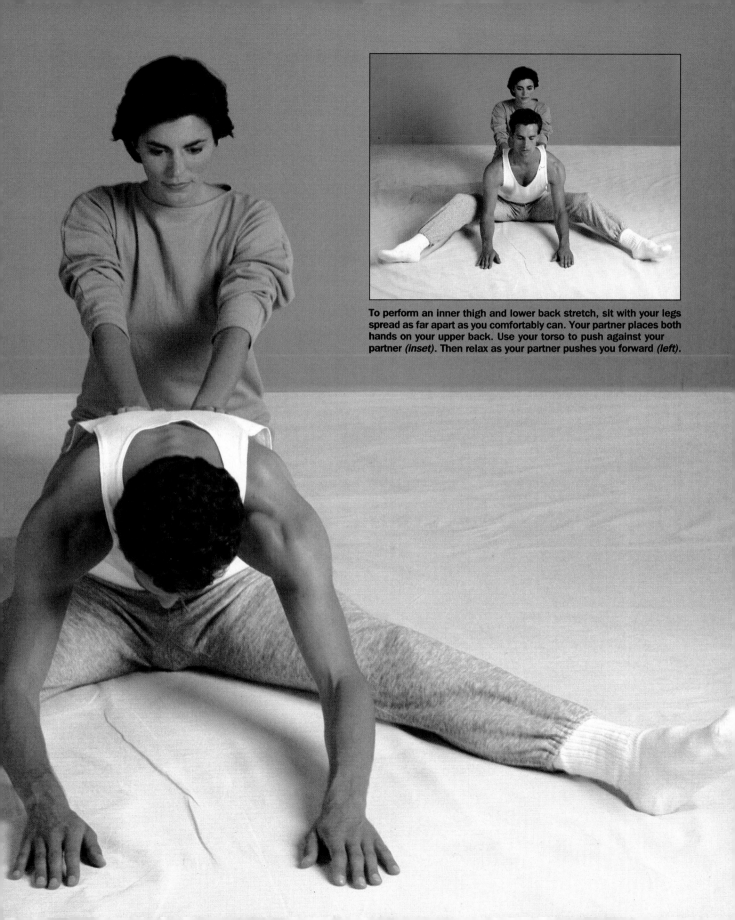

To perform an inner thigh and lower back stretch, sit with your legs spread as far apart as you comfortably can. Your partner places both hands on your upper back. Use your torso to push against your partner *(inset)*. Then relax as your partner pushes you forward *(left)*.

# Quadriceps and Hip Flexors/1

The quadriceps and hip flexors are the primary muscles along the front of your thigh. They are extremely powerful and therefore lend themselves particularly well to partner-assisted routines, since your partner can use your leg as leverage.

If you run, cycle or climb stairs frequently, you should also stretch the iliotibial band, a strip of connective tissue that runs from one of the hip flexors on the outside of your hip all the way down to the outside of your knee. The iliotibial can become tight from these activities and cause a burning sensation around the knee. The stretch on pages 66-67 is designed to loosen the iliotibial band.

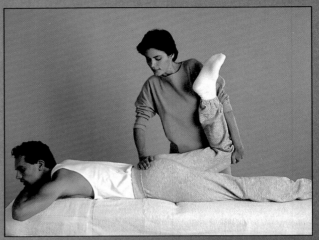

To isolate your hip flexors, lie face down on a table as your partner presses one hand against your right pelvis, grasps your right leg just above the knee and lifts it into a stretch.

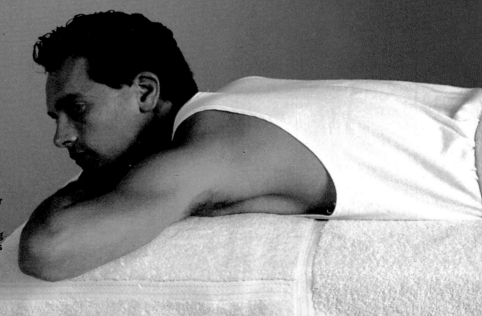

To perform a quadriceps stretch, lie face down on the floor or a massage table. Your partner stabilizes your pelvis with one hand and bends your leg with the other. Attempt to straighten your knee by pushing against her hand, then relax as she bends your leg to a new point of tightness.

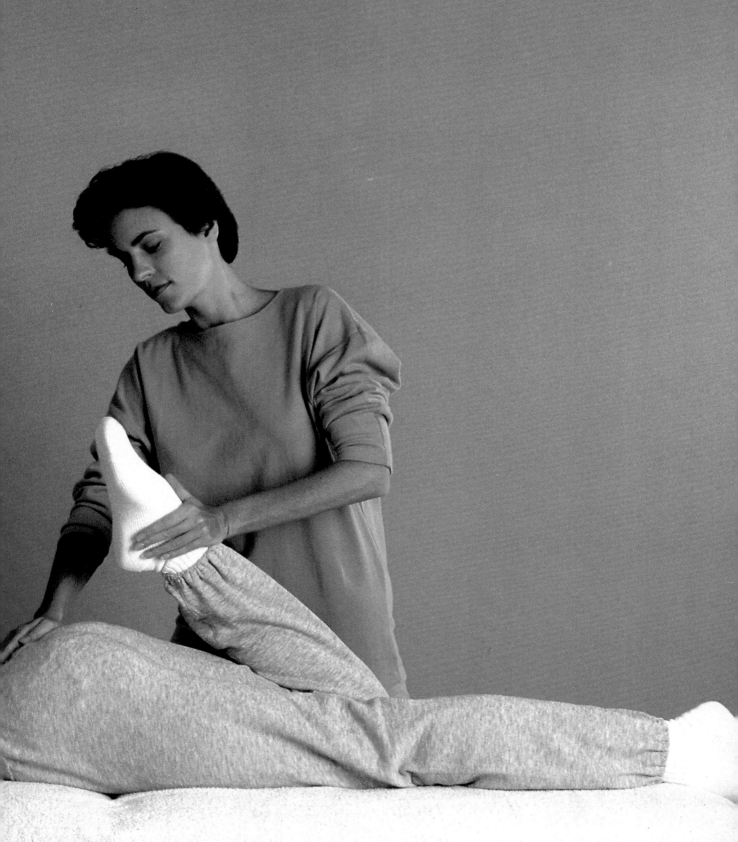

# Quadriceps and
# Hip Flexors/2

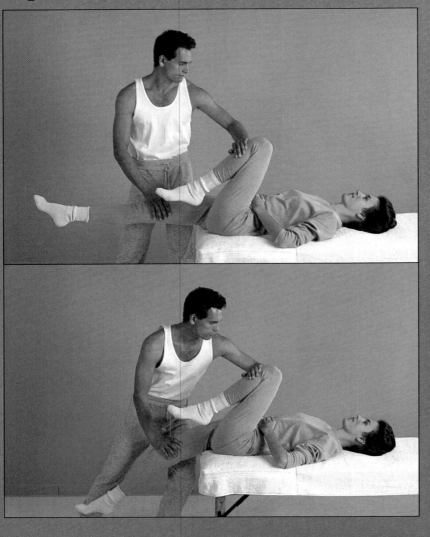

For an additional hip-flexor stretch, lie on your back with your buttocks near the end of a table. Stretch your right leg out and draw your left leg up *(top left)*. Your partner helps hold your left leg in place as you extend your right leg. Relax as your partner pushes your right leg down and your left knee toward your chest *(bottom left)*.

To loosen the iliotibial band, lie on your side at the end of a table. Bend the bottom leg to support your pelvis but keep your other leg straight. Your partner uses one hand to hold your pelvis and the other hand to press down lightly on your knee *(right)*.

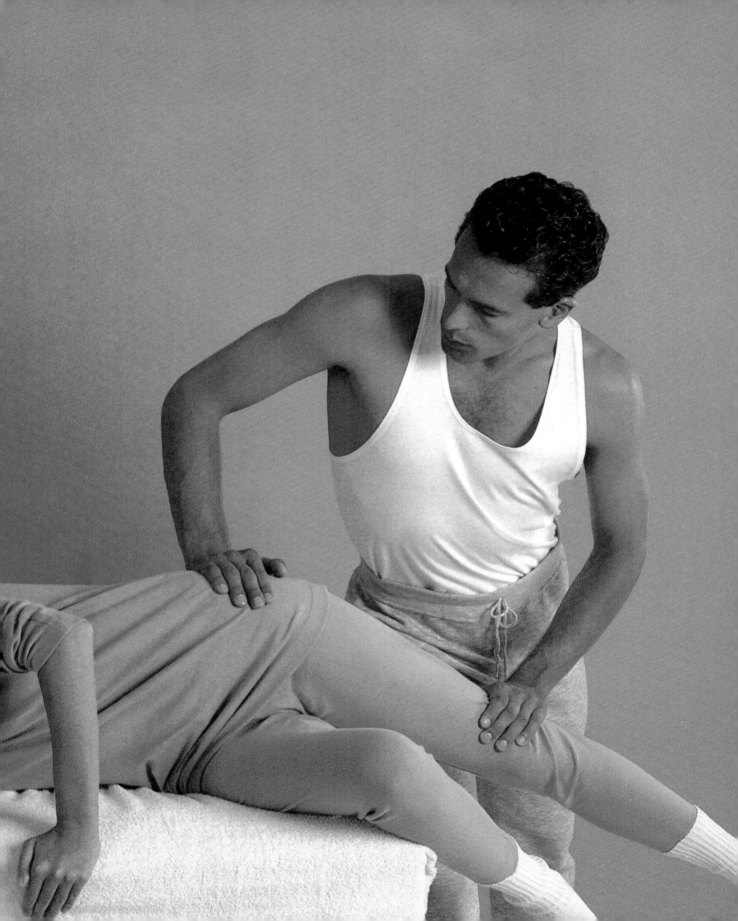

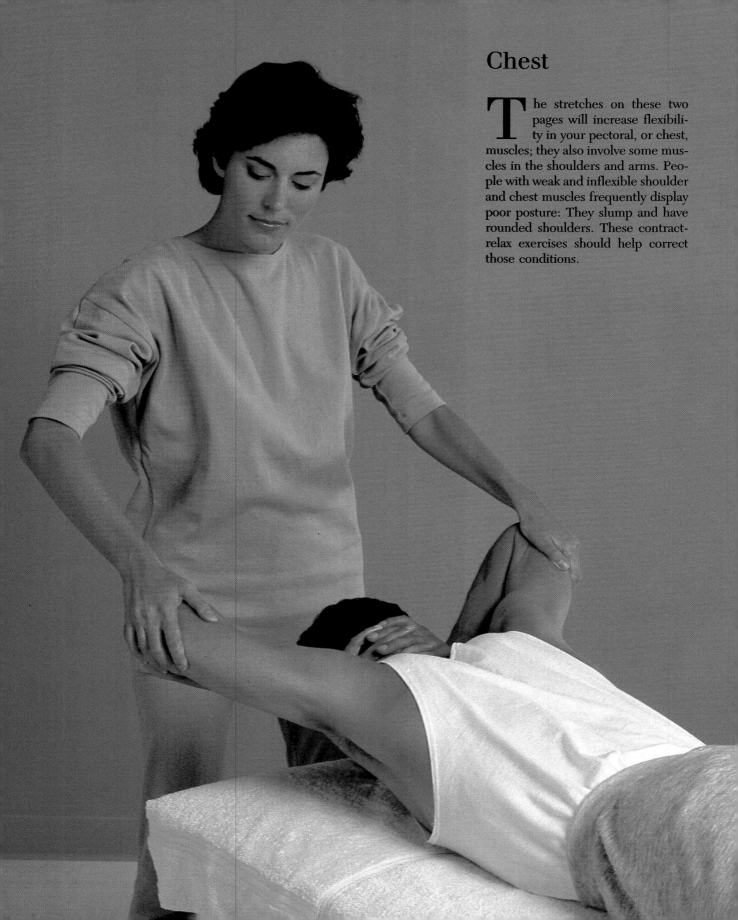

# Chest

The stretches on these two pages will increase flexibility in your pectoral, or chest, muscles; they also involve some muscles in the shoulders and arms. People with weak and inflexible shoulder and chest muscles frequently display poor posture: They slump and have rounded shoulders. These contract-relax exercises should help correct those conditions.

Lie face down on a table. As your partner draws your arms up by the wrists, the force of your body weight stretches your chest muscles. Keep your elbows loose.

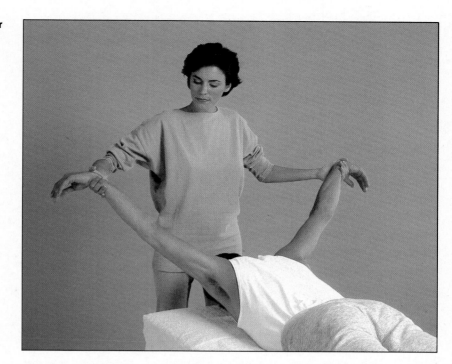

Sit cross-legged with your back supported by your partner's leg. Interlace your fingers behind your head. Your partner pulls your elbows back.

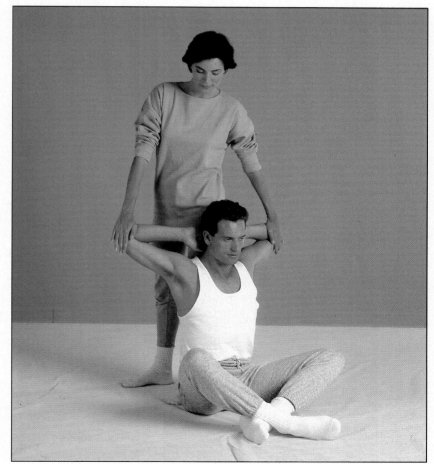

Lie face down on a table with your hands clasped behind your head *(opposite)*. Your partner grasps your elbows and draws them up. You will feel a stretch of the pectorals of the chest and the biceps and triceps of the upper arm.

# Back

**Y**our back contains dozens of muscles in five crisscrossing layers. The outer layer consists of the latissimus dorsi and the trapezius, both of which influence shoulder movement. Most of the inner layers of back muscles are anchored on your pelvis and are connected to your vertebrae and ribs. These muscles hold your spinal column erect and permit your spine to move in all directions; they allow you to rotate around and arch backward, forward and sideways. Despite their importance, these muscles are often too short and easily strained, causing backache. Partner-assisted back stretches help provide gentle traction and stretch these deep spinal muscles.

**To stretch the muscles of the upper back and chest, kneel and extend your hands in front of you while pressing your chest downward. Your partner overlaps her hands and presses gently on your spine.**

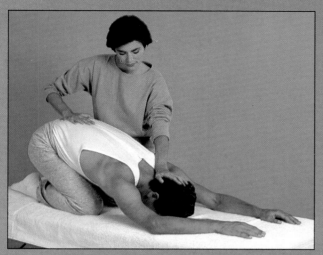

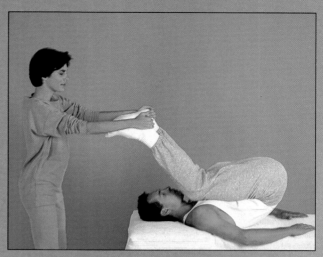

To stretch the entire spine, assume a kneeling position, lean over and sit back on your heels. Your partner places her hands on your head and lower back. Without moving her hands, she exerts pressure gently but firmly in opposite directions *(above)*.

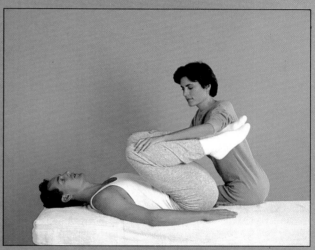

To stretch the lower back, buttocks and hamstrings, lie on your back and draw your legs up *(top)*. Your partner grasps your ankles and pulls them over your head. To stretch just the lower back and buttocks *(above)*, your partner pushes your knees to your chest.

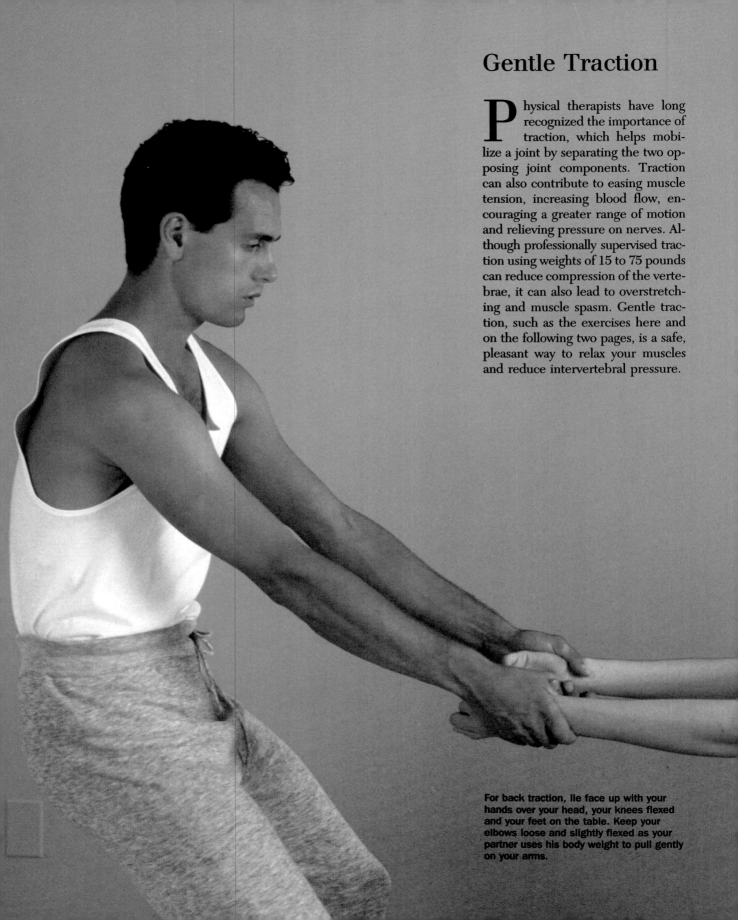

# Gentle Traction

Physical therapists have long recognized the importance of traction, which helps mobilize a joint by separating the two opposing joint components. Traction can also contribute to easing muscle tension, increasing blood flow, encouraging a greater range of motion and relieving pressure on nerves. Although professionally supervised traction using weights of 15 to 75 pounds can reduce compression of the vertebrae, it can also lead to overstretching and muscle spasm. Gentle traction, such as the exercises here and on the following two pages, is a safe, pleasant way to relax your muscles and reduce intervertebral pressure.

For back traction, lie face up with your hands over your head, your knees flexed and your feet on the table. Keep your elbows loose and slightly flexed as your partner uses his body weight to pull gently on your arms.

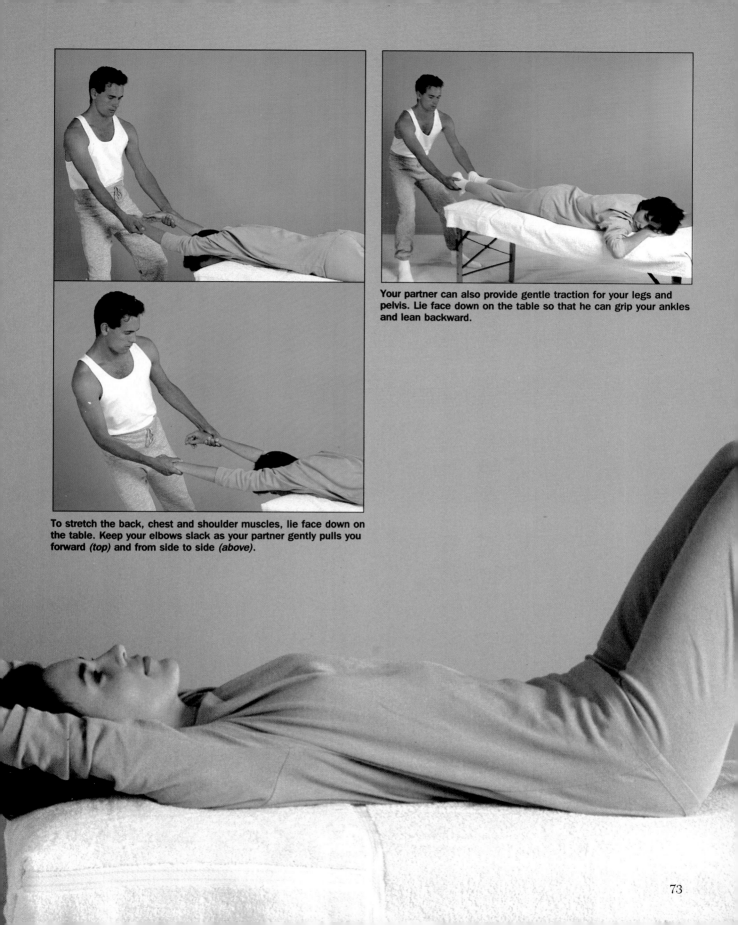

Your partner can also provide gentle traction for your legs and pelvis. Lie face down on the table so that he can grip your ankles and lean backward.

To stretch the back, chest and shoulder muscles, lie face down on the table. Keep your elbows slack as your partner gently pulls you forward *(top)* and from side to side *(above)*.

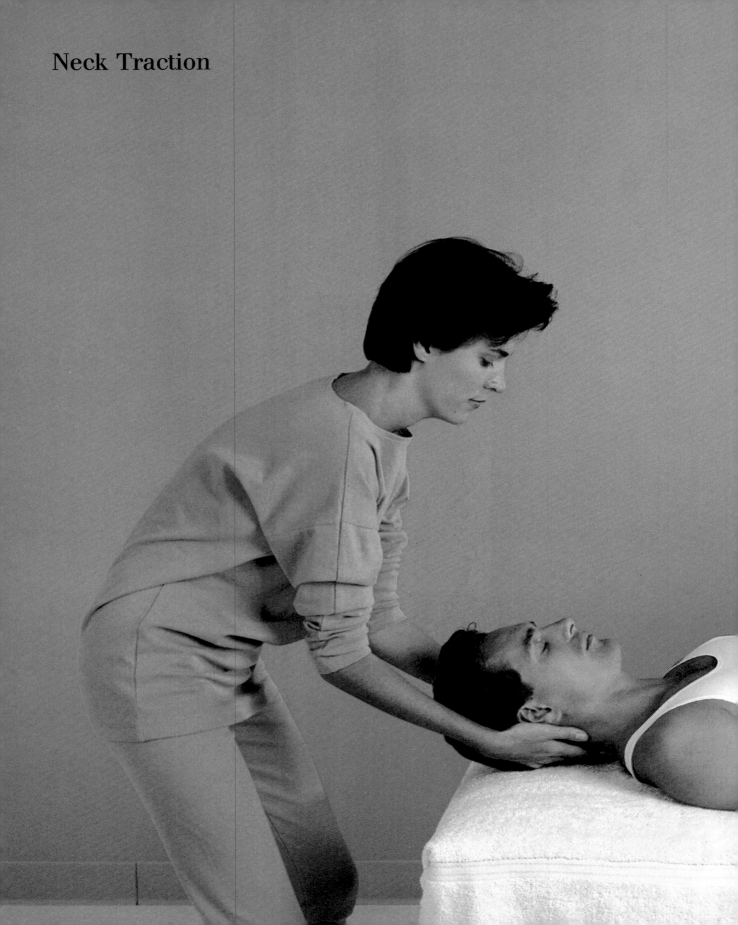

# Neck Traction

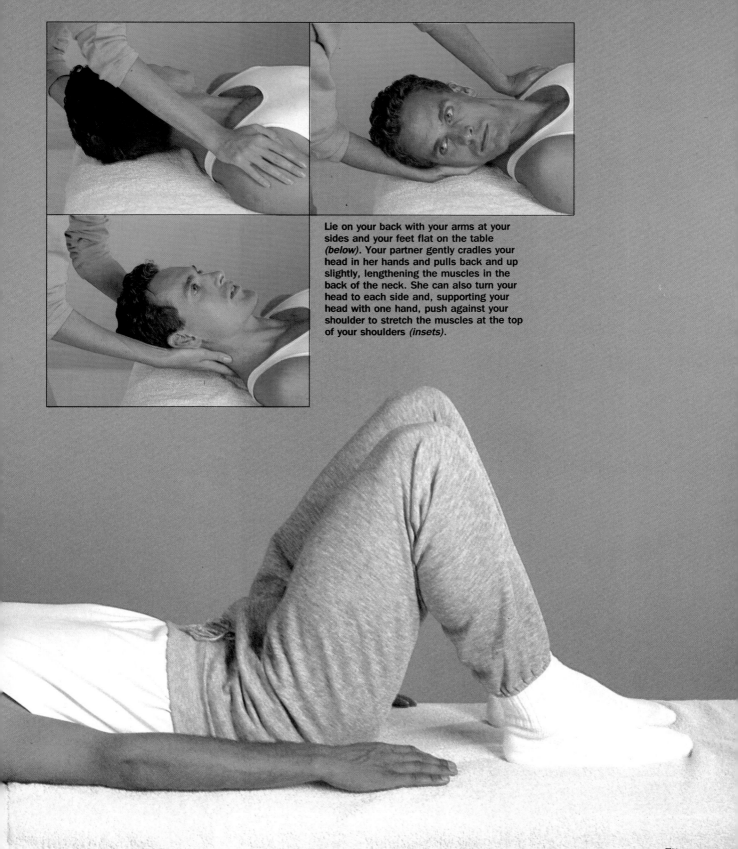

Lie on your back with your arms at your sides and your feet flat on the table *(below)*. Your partner gently cradles your head in her hands and pulls back and up slightly, lengthening the muscles in the back of the neck. She can also turn your head to each side and, supporting your head with one hand, push against your shoulder to stretch the muscles at the top of your shoulders *(insets)*.

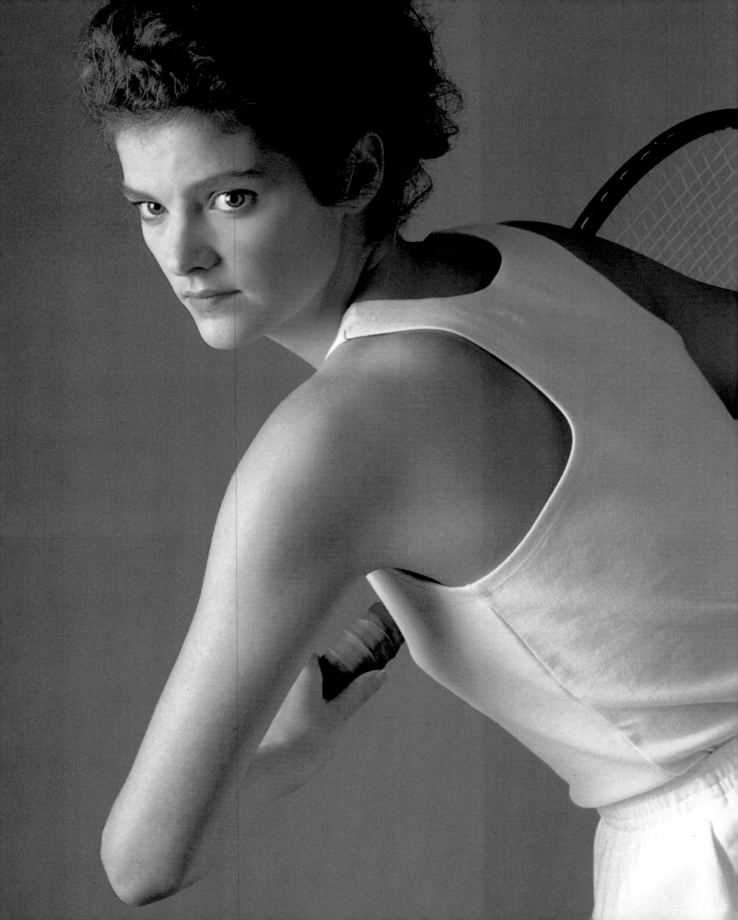

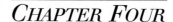

# CHAPTER FOUR

# Stretching for Sports

*Better performance,
fewer injuries*

T o most athletes, the benefits of
stretching and good flexibility are obvious. A full range of motion in
certain joints is necessary for the successful performance of many
sports. Dance, figure skating and gymnastics, for example, require
extensive muscular flexibility and a good range of motion in virtually
all body joints. Contact sports like football, hockey, basketball and
soccer also require a better-than-average range of motion in the joints,
as well as flexibility in the muscles of the thigh, hip flexors, trunk,
arms, shoulders and neck. For most noncontact sports like track and
field, swimming, golf and baseball, you need varying degrees of flexibility specific to the particular sport. For example, swimmers who
perform the front crawl will especially benefit from improved flexibility in the rotator cuff muscles of the shoulders. Without it, they may
experience limitations in their stroking ability and possibly develop a
stress injury called swimmer's shoulder.

Flexibility is also related to power. Experiments have shown that muscles can store elastic energy and then release that energy in a powerful burst. The more a muscle can stretch, the greater its potential for energy release during contraction. Thus, muscle elasticity plays an important role in sports that require forceful stretch and contraction, such as jumping and throwing. Baseball pitchers, for instance, need to be especially flexible in the chest. Like the string of a bow, the major chest muscle is pulled taut as the arm swings back to pitch a ball; like an arrow, the farther the ball is drawn back, the more force can be applied to it and the greater its velocity when released.

Runners, too, may be able to improve their performance by increasing their flexibility. According to a U.S. Olympic track coach, tight muscles present internal resistance to movement. Runners with loose, pliant leg muscles, therefore, may be able to move their legs faster and longer than those with tighter muscles. And by adding just an inch to your stride length through stretching, you can gain about seven yards per quarter mile. For such distance events as a 10,000-meter run or a 26.2-mile marathon, even a minuscule increase in stride length can make the difference between a world-class performance and simply finishing the race.

Coaches and athletes alike generally accept the importance of stretching and flexibility for the enhancement of sports performance. Although few studies have been conducted in the area of flexibility and performance, there is some evidence that increased flexibility can improve performance in certain specific activities such as long jumping, ball hitting, throwing and sprinting. No studies have established minimum norms of flexibility necessary for each sports activity, however; nor has research determined how general sports performance may change in response to a progressive stretching program.

While it is clear that some level of flexibility is essential for the successful performance of any sport, once you have reached that level, you may not be able to improve your performance further by continuing to increase flexibility. For example, slight variations in flexibility among a group of top gymnasts will not determine who will rank highest in competition. However, gymnasts and other athletes must stretch to achieve the level of flexibility required by their sport and continue stretching to maintain that flexibility.

Some studies suggest that stretching can also help prevent injuries. A study of Swedish soccer players showed that athletes with muscle tightness and restricted range of motion have a higher-than-average incidence of injuries. Muscle strains occurred in 31 percent of the players with muscle tightness, but in only 18 percent of the players with normal flexibility. Studies of soccer players in the United States show that those players with tight or inflexible hamstring muscles may develop lower back and knee injuries.

The reason for this is that muscles adapt to exercise by shortening to the range of motion habitually used in the exercise. And vigorous exercise places greater loads on inflexible muscles, leading to chronic stress injuries. A short gastrocnemius muscle in the calf, for instance,

## Hand Stretches

Your hands are crucial tools for playing almost any sport. First, they translate muscle power from your body into the motion of a racquet, ball or club. They must also control that motion, giving a precise arc to a basketball, for instance, or the right angle and velocity to a tennis shot. In addition, your hands may have to support your body, such as during a long cycling trip.

Use the four simple exercises at right to stretch your hands for power and flexibility. The top two are for your thumbs, the bottom two for your fingers. Before you perform them, shake your hands vigorously to increase circulation.

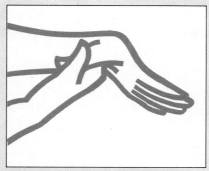

Firmly but gently stretch your thumb toward your wrist. Do not force it.

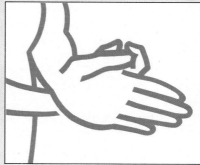

Stretch your thumb in the opposite direction by pulling back on it.

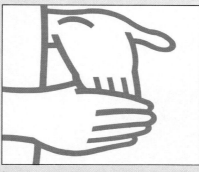

Stretch your palm by pulling back on all your fingers at the same time.

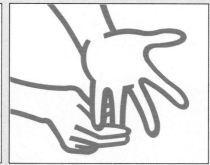

Spread your fingers and pull them back one at a time.

may result in pronation, or inward rotation of the foot, which is the most common cause of stress injuries to the foot and can lead to ankle and leg injuries and even a stress fracture.

If you do get an injury, stretching may help you recover more easily: It has been shown to reduce muscle soreness, and many athletes believe that it also speeds recovery. In addition, muscle injury often results in the formation of scar tissue, which is inelastic and acts to reduce a muscle's pliability. Thus, stretching exercises can help restore flexibility to an injured muscle.

Since flexibility is muscle-specific — that is, you become more flexible only in the muscles you stretch — and each sport places its own pattern of stress on joints and other body parts, your stretching routine must vary according to which sports you play. The following 16 pages offer stretching routines for eight of the most often played recreational sports. These routines will not necessarily make you a better player, but they can keep you from getting injured and enhance your enjoyment of the game.

# Baseball

Almost everyone, whatever his level of conditioning, can enjoy a good game of baseball. Nevertheless, it helps if you have agility and coordination and can muster explosive bursts of strength and speed for pitching, batting and running. To prepare for such bursts and to protect yourself from possible injury, you should stretch out frequently, particularly if you play baseball often.

Perform the lunge at right to stretch the hip flexors of the straight leg and the buttocks muscles of the bent leg. Feel the stretch in the shoulders, the upper back and the latissimus dorsi. Assume a sitting position with arms extended (inset) to stretch your inner thighs and lower back.

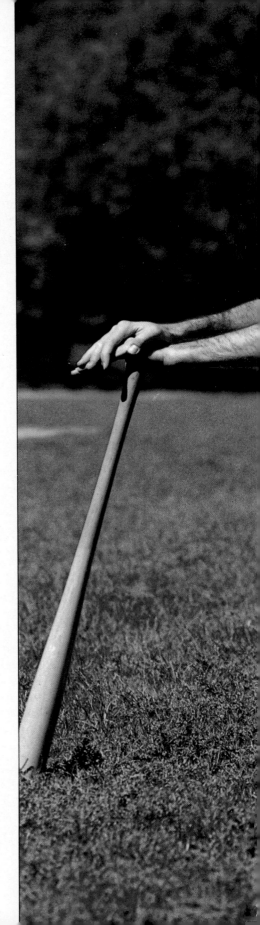

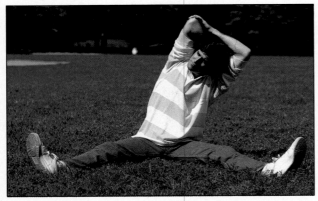

Grasp your elbows over your head and pull to one side to stretch your latissimus dorsi, chest, obliques and side muscles.

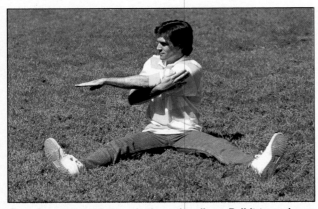

Extend one arm and grasp it above the elbow. Pull it toward your chest to stretch your shoulder and middle back muscles.

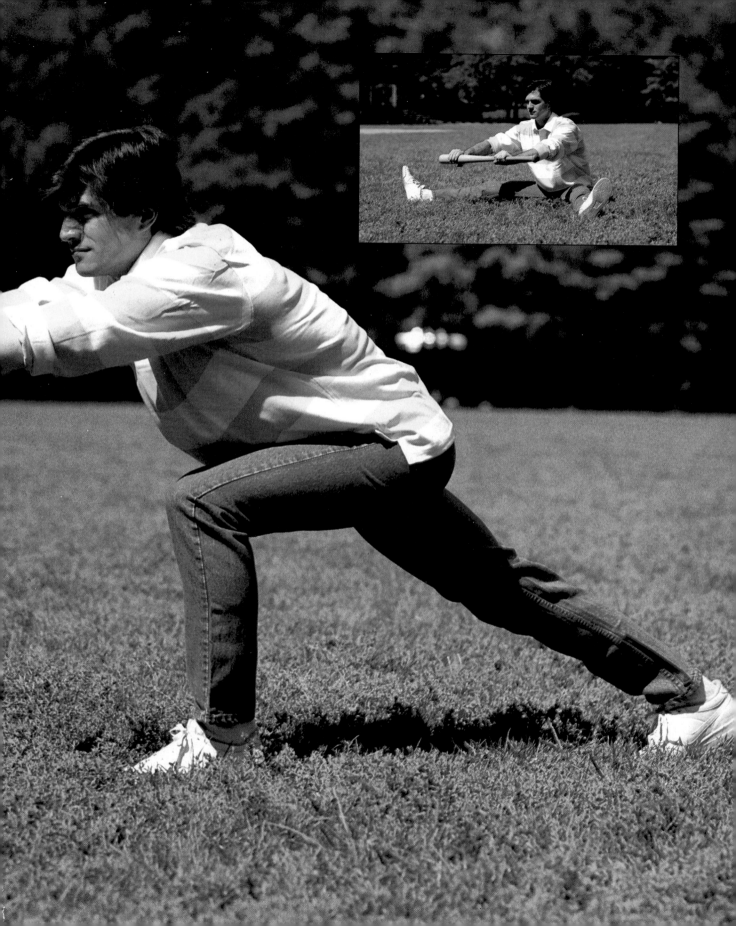

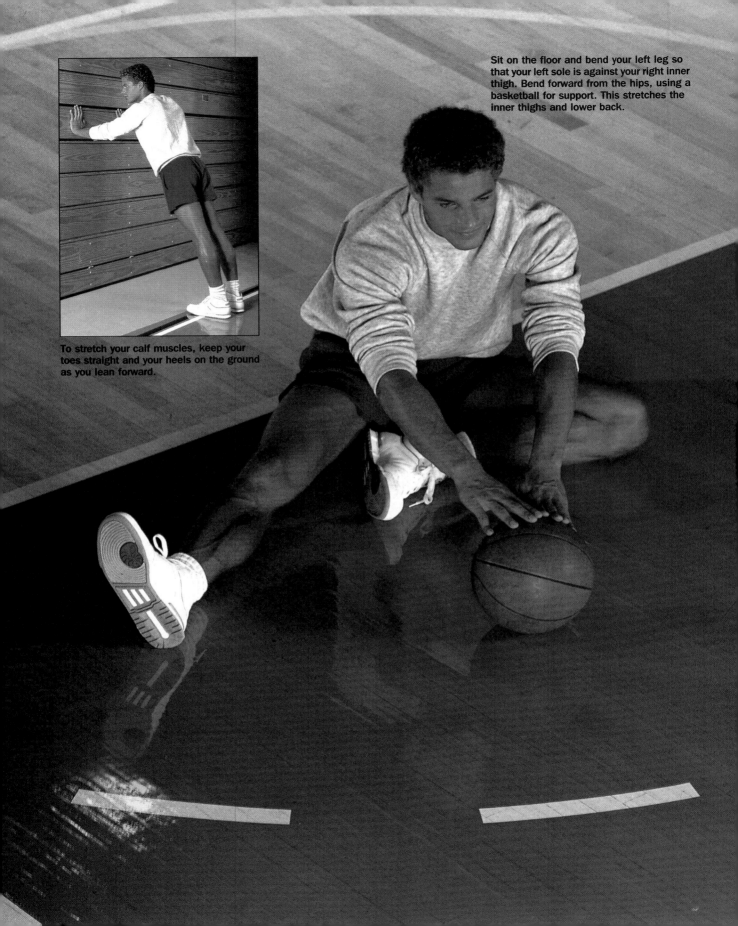

Sit on the floor and bend your left leg so that your left sole is against your right inner thigh. Bend forward from the hips, using a basketball for support. This stretches the inner thighs and lower back.

To stretch your calf muscles, keep your toes straight and your heels on the ground as you lean forward.

# Basketball

**B**asketball is a sport that requires not only coordination and agility, but a great deal of stamina, jumping ability and speed. Basketball is a fast, stop-and-start sport that involves twisting and turning and sudden dashes and leaps on a hard court surface. In addition, basketball unavoidably involves occasional collisions.

Basketball players need strength and flexibility, particularly in their hips, thighs, calves and trunk. These two pages present six basic stretches that will help loosen you up to play basketball. These stretches focus particular attention on the hip region, which is where most of the stress of basketball's demanding twists and turns occurs.

While sitting, draw one knee up. Extend your arms and lean forward from the hips to stretch the hamstrings of the straight leg.

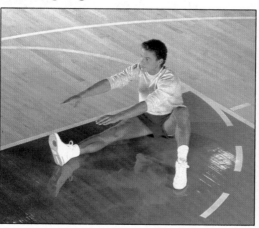

Remain seated and cross your legs, pulling your right knee toward your chest. You will feel the stretch in your right buttocks.

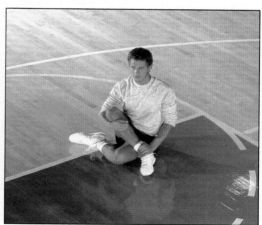

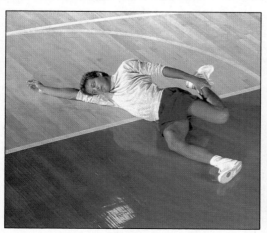

Lie on your right side and extend your right arm. Pull your left foot toward your buttocks but keep your knee in line with your hip to stretch your quadriceps.

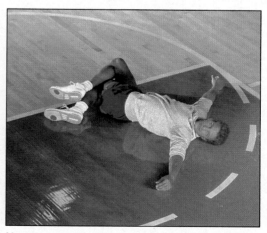

Lie on your back with your arms outstretched. Twist your legs to the right. Cross your right leg over your left to stretch the outer hip, thigh and lower back.

# Bicycling

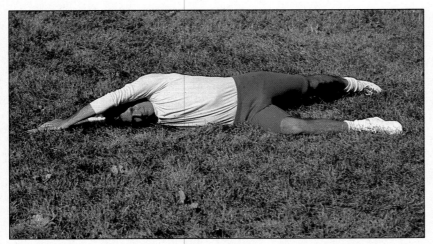

Lie on your back and extend your legs into the air, keeping your knees straight. Support your legs with your hands and separate them to stretch the inner thighs.

Lie on your right side with both arms extended as shown. Draw your left leg back until you feel a stretch in the hip flexors, outer thighs and latissimus dorsi.

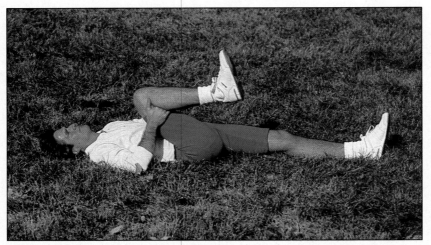

Lie on your back and draw your right knee toward your chest. Use your arms to pull the back of your knee. You should feel a stretch in the hip flexors and lower back.

**B**icycling is an endurance sport that requires as much effort and stamina as long-distance running. As in running, the great muscles of the calves and thighs provide most of the driving force needed to propel you forward. Cycling requires particular flexibility and strength in the hip flexors to draw the pedals up and, similarly, in the quadriceps to push the pedals down. For this reason, good cyclists have unusually powerful and pliant thigh muscles.

Because cycling places such a demand on the musculature of the legs and trunk, endurance riding all too often leads to muscle strain and pain in the lower back. These discomforts occur in novices and seasoned cyclists alike. In addition, cyclists often suffer from neck stiffness and sore wrists. For neck soreness, turn to pages 52-53; otherwise, the five stretches presented on these two pages should be all you need to help you maintain flexibility for bicycling.

Find an object just below waist level for support. Clasp your hands behind your head and place one foot on the object *(opposite)*. Keep your back straight and your heel on the ground to stretch the hip flexors, calf, Achilles tendon, chest and buttocks. Perform the stretch at right *(inset)* for the wrist flexors, shins and ankles. With your wrists reversed, lean forward as shown: Bending your right knee will stretch the ankle and shin in your left leg extending behind.

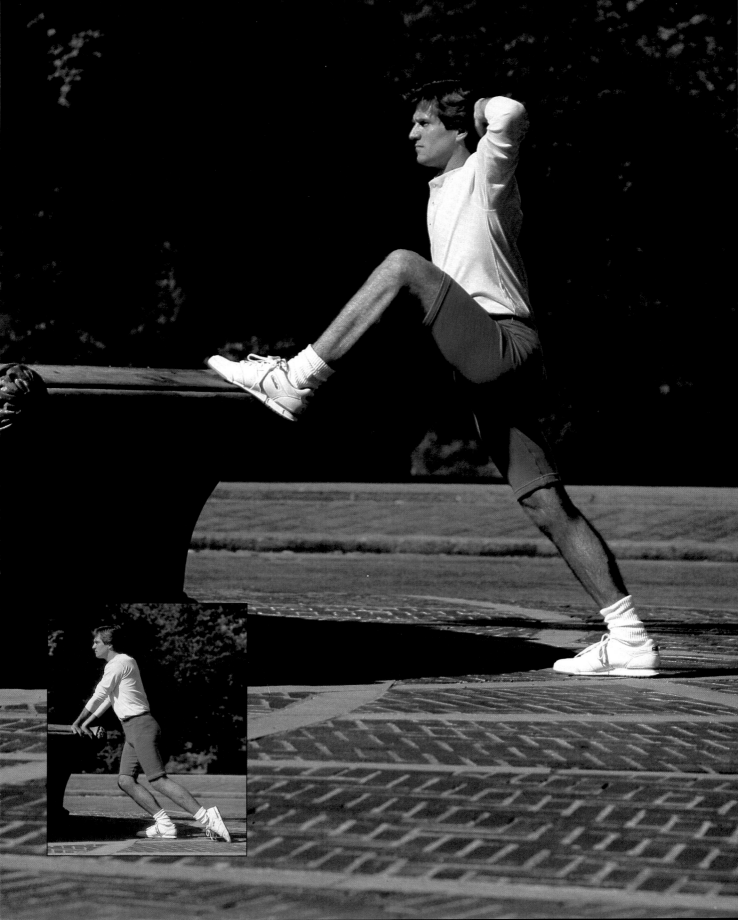

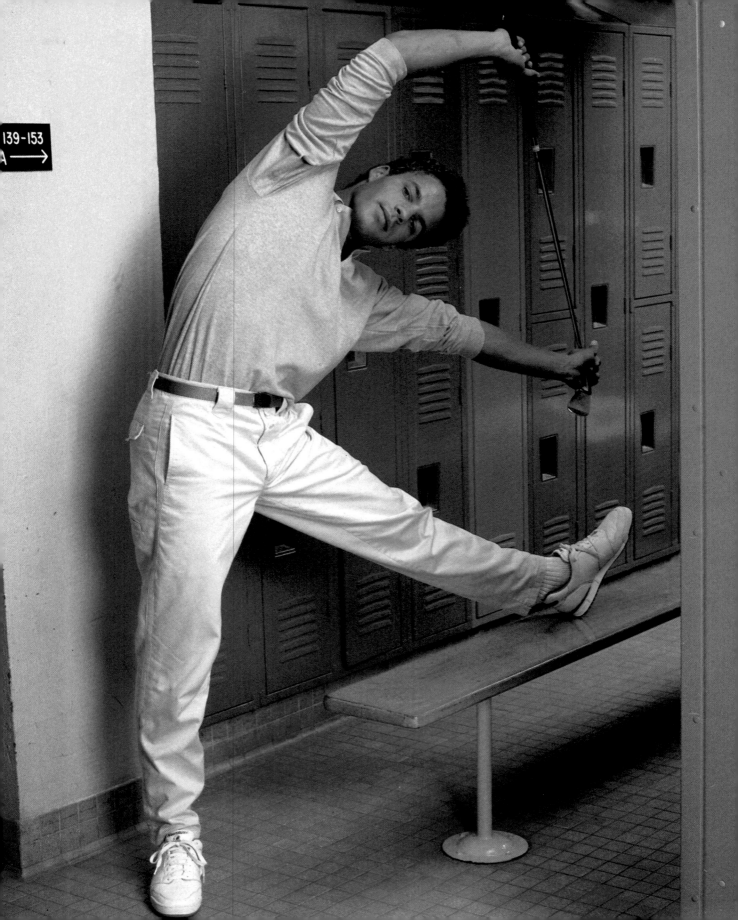

139-153
A ⟶

# Golf

Golf is a popular weekend sport; yet most people neglect the fitness aspects of the game. Golf requires a good deal more strength and endurance than most golfers realize, especially for those who carry their own golf clubs. Many weekend golfers also fail to appreciate the importance of fitness for improving their game and preventing injuries. A good golf swing involves a powerful twist of the arms, spine and shoulders in order to bring the head of the club around with sufficient force. In addition, the momentum of the club carries the golfer's arms into a wide arc, which may cause strains and even tears in the muscles of the shoulders, back, sides and wrists.

To minimize the chance of injury, and to give yourself the greatest range of motion in the joints of the shoulders and upper body, perform these four stretches.

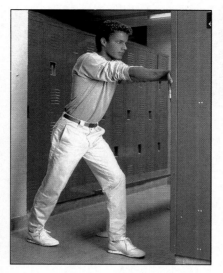

**Place your palms against a wall with your fingers pointing down. Move one leg forward while keeping the other leg straight. Lean into the wall. This not only stretches your calf, Achilles tendon and wrist flexors, but should also help you avoid golfer's elbow, an inflammation of the connective tissue in the elbow.**

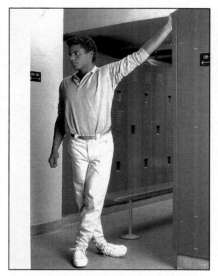

**Turn sideways to a wall and support yourself with your left arm. Swing your right leg behind your left and lean on the outside of the foot, twisting your body to produce a stretch in your left chest. This will also stretch the outer muscles of the right leg.**

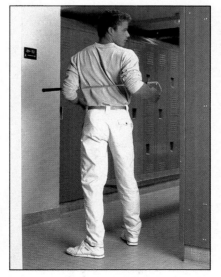

**To improve flexibility in your spine, place your golf club behind your back and under the inside of your elbows. Then turn your head to the right and twist your body to the right from the waist up.**

**Extend one leg to the side and rest it on a bench or stool** *(opposite)*. **Grasping your golf club at each end and holding it above your head, bend sideways toward the extended foot. You will be stretching the latissimus dorsi, the obliques and the inner thigh of the opposite leg.**

# Racquet Sports

Racquet sports, which include badminton, squash, racquetball and tennis, are excellent all-around conditioners. However, these sports are performed most frequently by recreational players who pay little attention to the fitness aspects of the activities. Most players launch right into their games with little or no warm-up, play intensely for a short period of time and then stop playing abruptly, only to resume days or weeks later. The consequence is almost inevitably injury. Few realize how physically demanding these sports can be, nor how much their game could improve if they simply took a little time to get into better condition. One of the best ways to improve your condition and to avoid unnecessary injuries is to improve your flexibility.

Racquet sports require speed and agility, particularly for quick lateral movements. Thus, players with tight muscles may experience frequent groin muscle pulls. And since returning a ball in play often calls for sudden lunges and stretches, pulls in the back, sides, wrist, ankles and shoulders are also common. These two pages offer five stretches to help you improve your racquet game.

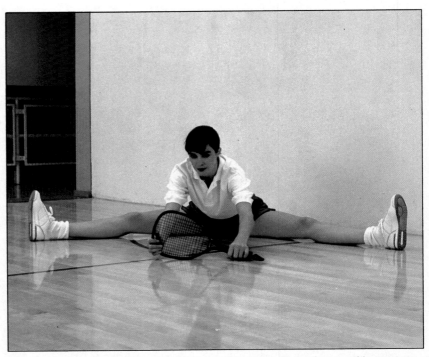

Sit on the floor with your knees straight but not locked and your feet as wide apart as comfortably possible. Hold your racquet on the floor in front of you for support; lean forward from the waist. You should feel a stretch of your inner thighs, lower back and upper back.

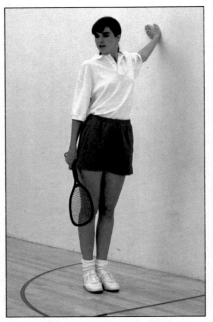

To stretch your chest muscles, stand at arm's length from a wall and place one palm on the wall as shown. Turn your body slightly away from the wall but keep your hand in place.

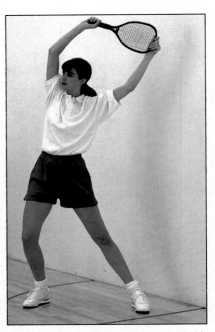

Grasp both ends of your racquet and hold it over your head. Spread your feet apart and arc your body to the left, bending your right knee slightly but keeping your left leg straight.

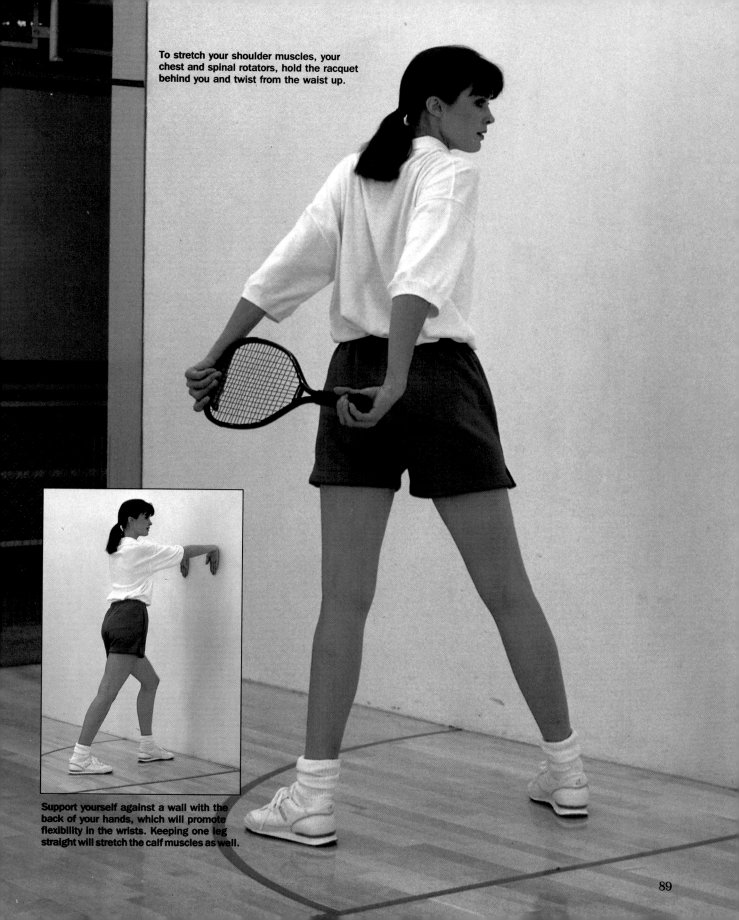

To stretch your shoulder muscles, your chest and spinal rotators, hold the racquet behind you and twist from the waist up.

Support yourself against a wall with the back of your hands, which will promote flexibility in the wrists. Keeping one leg straight will stretch the calf muscles as well.

89

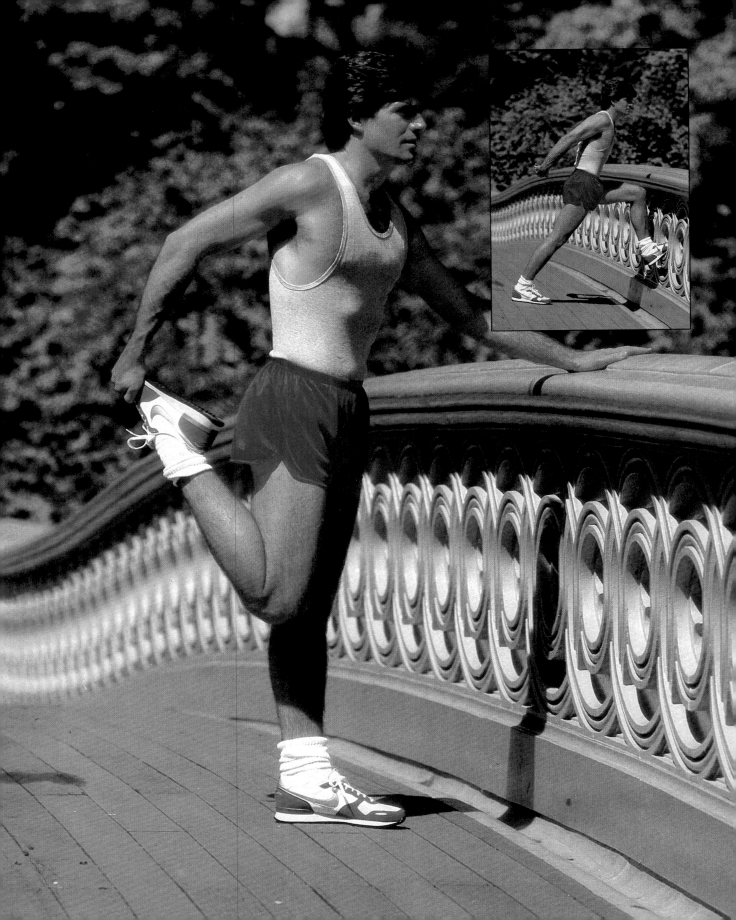

# Running

**R**unning is probably the most efficient way to get into shape. Almost anyone can run at almost any time and with a minimum of expense. Studies show that virtually anyone can increase cardiovascular fitness with running, including children, the elderly and even heart attack victims. No wonder, then, that millions of Americans run on a regular basis.

Running, however, places great stress on the body's muscles and tendons. According to one survey, about half a sample population of runners reported a running injury in the previous year that was serious enough to make them reduce training, take medication or see a health professional. A disproportionate percentage of running injuries occurs among beginning joggers who have not developed adequate strength or flexibility.

To avoid injury and increase your range of motion for running, thereby promoting a more fluid running style, you should perform the stretches on these two pages.

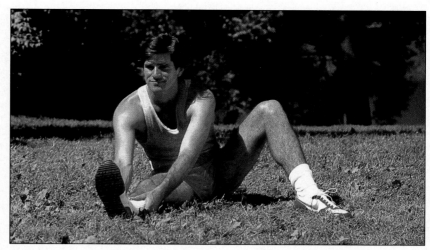

Sit on the ground and draw your left knee up. Lean forward from the hips and reach for your right ankle to stretch the hamstrings of the straight leg.

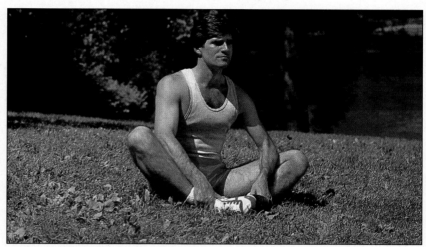

Draw the soles of your feet together and clasp your ankles for support. Lean forward slightly from the hips to stretch your inner thighs and lower back.

**To stretch the quadriceps, hold onto an object for balance, pull your right heel back toward your right buttocks *(left)* and keep your knee pointing toward the ground. Stretch your hip flexors, calves, shoulders and chest by clasping your hands behind your back and placing your left foot on an object about a foot off the ground *(inset)*. Keep your right knee straight, lean forward and pull your arms up.**

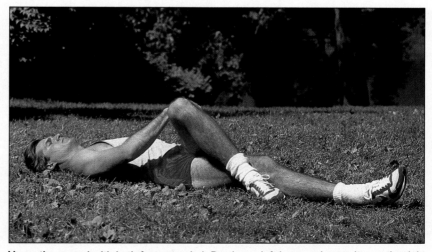

Lie on the ground with both feet extended. Bend your left knee and cross it over the right leg. Pull your knee toward the ground to stretch the muscles of the outer hip and thigh.

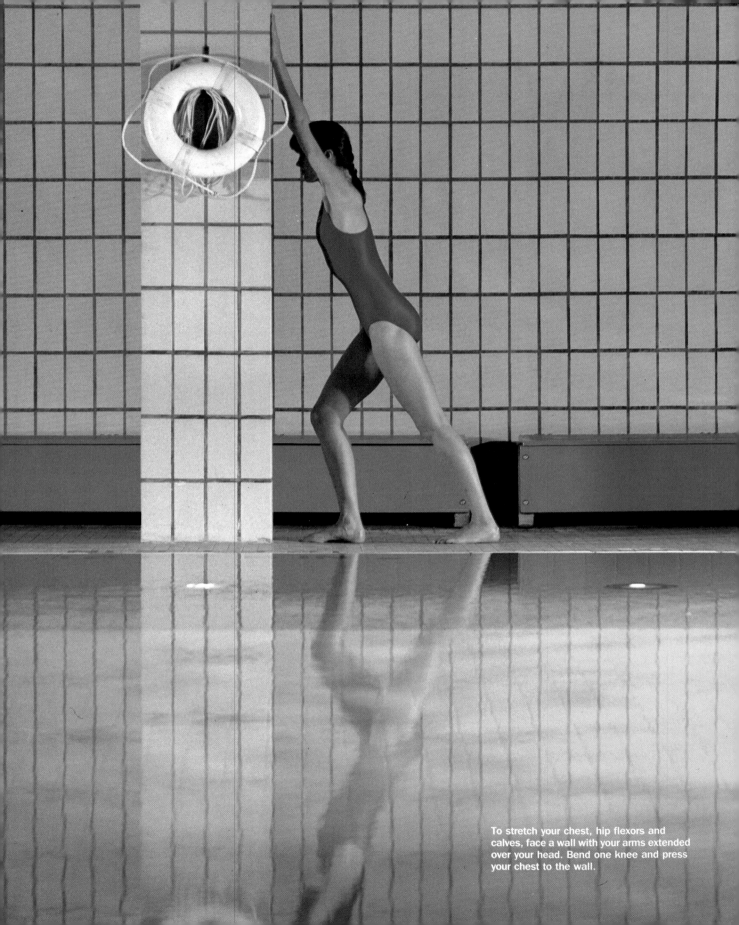

To stretch your chest, hip flexors and calves, face a wall with your arms extended over your head. Bend one knee and press your chest to the wall.

# Swimming

Swimming is one of the most popular sports in the United States. Although you do not have to be particularly skillful or fit to enjoy swimming, this activity can place a tremendous demand on virtually all of your body's major muscle groups. Swimmers need strong arms, shoulders, chests and abdomens, since the muscles grouped in those areas provide most of your stroking power. Because swimming is a dynamic sport that requires full range of motion, particularly in the shoulders, you must stretch out frequently to avoid tight muscles. Perform the six stretches on these two pages at least once a day.

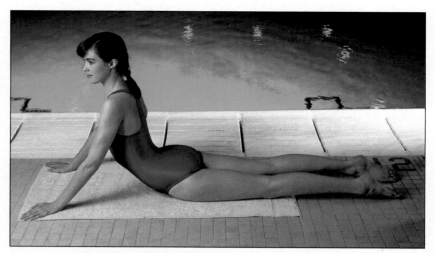

Lie on your stomach and extend your arms, keeping your hips on the floor. You will feel the stretch in your abdominals and hip flexors.

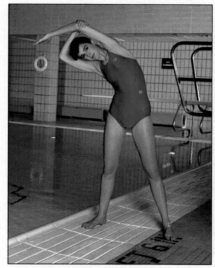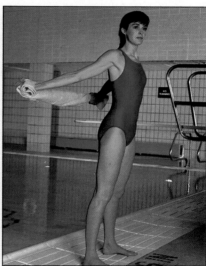

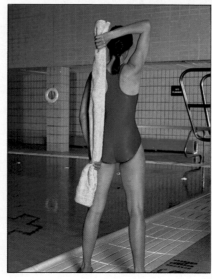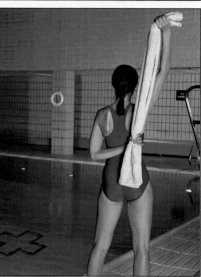

Stand with your arms above your head and grasp your left elbow with your right hand. Pull your arm to the right *(top left)* to stretch the latissimus dorsi and obliques. For your shoulders and biceps *(top right)*, grasp a towel behind your back and pull it up with both arms. You can then use the towel to stretch the shoulder's rotator cuff muscles *(near right)*. Hold it behind your back and pull down with one arm while the other arm is just behind your head *(far right)*. Then pull up with one hand over your head while the other is bent behind your back.

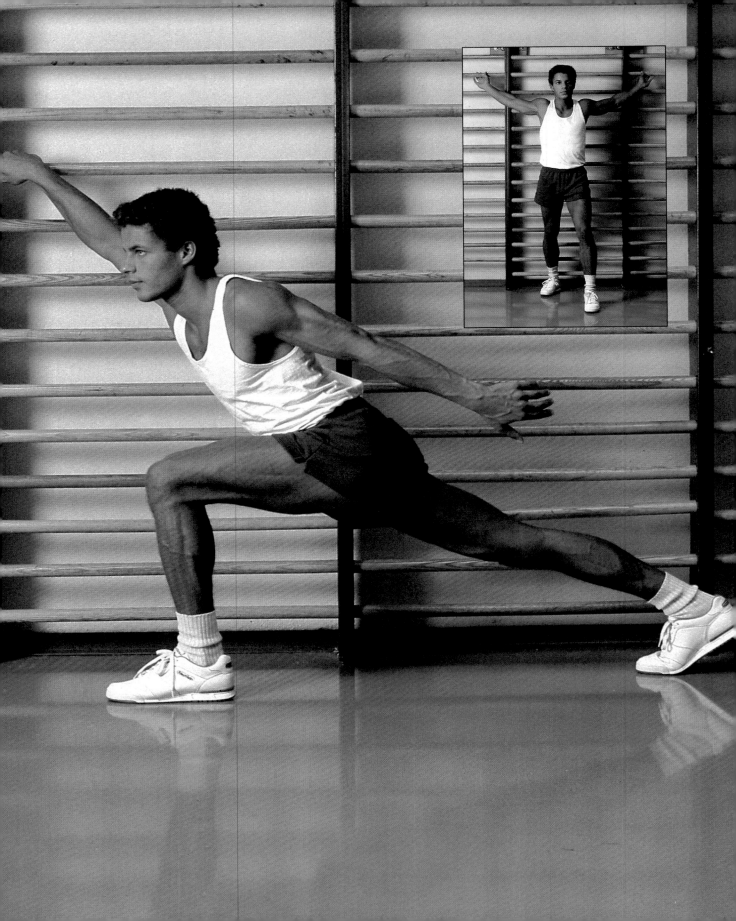

# Volleyball

Volleyball is a game conducted at a fast pace. It requires frequent bursts of speed and the ability to jump high and hit hard. Volleyball players need flexible shoulders and calves for spiking — smashing a ball downward from the top of a jump. Supple hip flexors and inner thighs are also important so as not to pull a muscle when you drop down under the ball for a save.

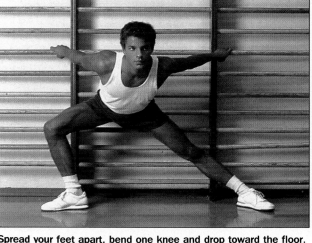

Spread your feet apart, bend one knee and drop toward the floor. Grasp a railing behind you with both hands and pull forward to stretch your chest, shoulders and inner thighs.

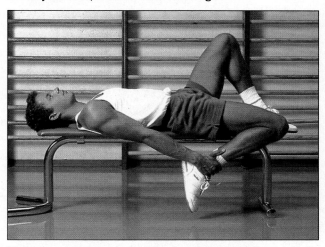

Lie face up, keeping your back flat by raising your left knee. Pull back on your right ankle for a quadriceps stretch.

To stretch the hip flexors and buttocks, perform a lunge *(left)*. You may hold on to an object such as a railing for support. For chest and shoulder muscles *(inset)*, grasp a railing behind you and lean forward. Place your right heel near the wall and bend your left knee to stretch your calves. Point your feet straight ahead and keep your heels down.

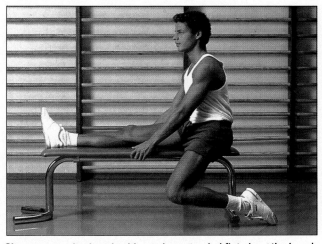

Sit on an exercise bench with one leg extended flat along the bench to stretch the hamstrings. Be sure to keep your back straight.

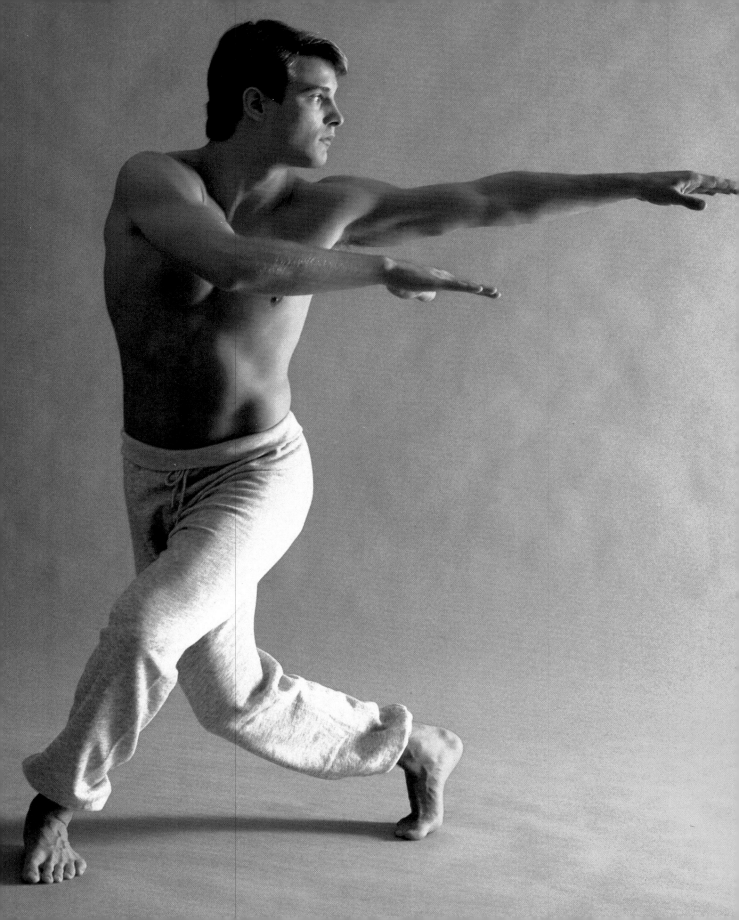

# CHAPTER FIVE

# Dynamic Movement

*A whole-body routine for fluid motion
in three dimensions*

In recent years, a new type of
exercise called dynamic movement has evolved, blending ancient
Eastern arts of movement with modern-day understanding of biomechanics, musculoskeletal anatomy and neuromuscular physiology. Its
reinterpretation of the lilting, dancelike forms of Tai Chi and the
deliberate actions of Yoga is aimed at enhancing body awareness,
freedom of movement, coordination and flexibility, and providing release from muscular tension.

From the perspective of dynamic movement, most conventional
stretching seems a one-dimensional activity. The action is most often
an up-and-down or back-and-forth motion perpendicular to the body,
and it ordinarily stretches a specific muscle or muscle group for a
particular activity. Recommended stretching exercises for runners, for
instance, elongate the muscles that get the most use: the calves,
hamstrings and hip flexors. Sometimes, to add a second dimension,
the athlete will stretch the muscles opposing the most-used muscles.

For the runner, these muscles are primarily the quadriceps along the front of the upper thigh.

Practitioners of dynamic movement think that this kind of stretching ignores a vital third dimension, the muscles that support the body as it moves. In daily life, they point out, we rarely move with the machine-like angularity implied by the one- or two-dimensional hamstrings-quadriceps stretching routine. Even the simplest action often requires the simultaneous involvement of numerous joints and the action of dozens, even hundreds, of muscles. Fluid body movement, therefore, can occur only as a result of intricate teamwork among groups of muscles acting sequentially.

Almost every movement involves properties of dynamic movement. Even if you try to stand still, your body does not remain motionless but sways slightly over a stationary base. Try as you may, you cannot stay absolutely still. Experiments show that people tend to faint when they are held absolutely still. Therefore, swaying slightly aids circulation and ensures continued consciousness. In order to continue this slight swaying yet not lose control, the body oscillates around a center line of gravity. Muscles and muscle groups all over the body alternately contract and relax. Even if you assume different positions or hold an object such as a book or a tray, your body automatically compensates and continues its oscillation. In dynamic movement, therefore, postural balance is seen as a fluctuation between stability and mobility.

Dynamic movement uses the stabilizing muscles that, when contracted, improve body stance and eliminate excessive movement that might occur as a body part moves. A stabilizing muscle keeps the area around it from moving so it can act as a fulcrum for other muscles to stretch and contract. This stabilizing action also prevents injury that might be caused by straining or by excessive stretching or compression of a joint. If you stand and then raise your right knee, the muscles most involved in lifting your knee are the right hip flexors. But the muscles that wrap around your right thighbone, for example, are also engaged, acting to guide the action and eliminate undesired rotary movements in the hip. The muscles in your trunk, pelvis and straight leg act to stabilize your body by alternately contracting and relaxing to maintain your position. While you are in motion, this type of force and counterforce occurs constantly in muscles all over your body, not just in the muscles most involved. It is impossible to understand running, for example, by viewing it simply as an action of the hip flexors, hamstrings and calves. It is a whole-body activity.

Exercise that involves the extra dimension provided by dynamic movement takes your body through various motions to lengthen and strengthen the supporting and assisting muscles. The first practitioners of dynamic movement, who were active in the 1920s and 1930s, used their exercises as a treatment to correct posture and alignment of the spine. In recent years, other disciplines like sports medicine and Yoga have enhanced the exercises, and practitioners in the field now work mainly with dancers to help them gain greater spatial

## The Kinesphere: The Body's Field of Movement

The body operates within a three-dimensional space. From a standing position, you can reach upward and downward, sideways and forward, backward and diagonally. You can also twist and turn around in the opposite direction. The space within your reach has length, width and depth. That space can be perceived as a sphere of movement: the kinesphere.

Unlike most traditional stretching and exercise routines, dynamic movement uses the entire space within your kinesphere. As you perform the dynamic movement routines shown on the following pages, you will become more aware of how your body movements function within this three-dimensional mode, not just in an up-and-down and back-and-forth action. Dynamic movement helps you realize your body's full, complex ranges of motion and the interrelationships of its various parts.

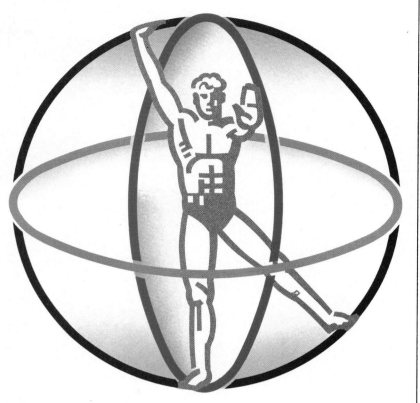

awareness through an understanding of body movements. There are several schools of dynamic movement, each named after a founder in the field; the best-known are Alexander, Laban and Feldenkrais. But although techniques vary from school to school, all of the exercises — including the ones in this chapter — are concerned with moving through combinations of lying, sitting and standing. Ultimately, the feelings of dynamic movement are those of ease and efficiency.

To begin your dynamic movement routines, find a well-ventilated room where you will not be interrupted or distracted. It should have a floor covering such as carpeting or matting to prevent discomfort while you are lying prone. Set aside plenty of time to perform your dynamic movement routines. Performing the routines hurriedly will destroy the sense of fluidity you are trying to develop.

Wear clothing that is appropriate for any type of stretching: Loose-fitting, nonbinding leotards or exercise outfits are perfect. Whatever you choose, do not wear a belt, which would restrict your movement and could become uncomfortable, or shoes, since there is no jumping activity that would pose a risk of foot injury.

# Preparing to Move

To get the most out of the dynamic movement exercises here and on the following pages, try to quiet your mind. Think of nothing but the physical act of moving. Never hurry through a movement or force yourself to attain a particular position. Do not perform a series of repetitions of the exercises rapidly, as if they were calisthenics; instead, move through an exercise slowly, with the poise and concentration of a dancer. Do each sequence two or three times during a session; they will soon become familiar and relaxing.

When you are performing a dynamic movement routine, be sure to breathe normally and rhythmically. Start each session by taking several deep breaths to help relax your entire system and keep breathing at a moderate pace. You should never force your breathing or constrict it.

As with more traditional stretching techniques, you should work both sides of your body equally. A routine that involves moving your body in one direction should be repeated in the other direction.

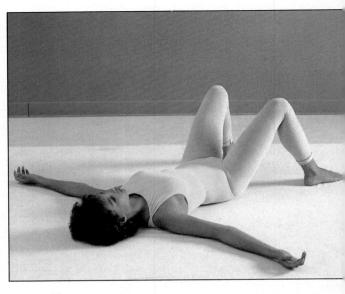

# Double-Arm Circle

**Lie face up on the floor with your knees bent and your arms outstretched** *(above)*. **Keeping your shoulders relaxed, slowly move your arms along the floor in an arc until they are over your head. Continue the circling movement until your arms cross, then lower them over your chest. Return to the starting position.**

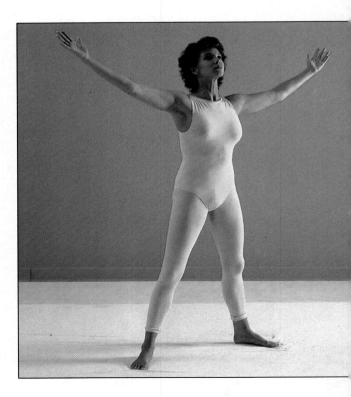

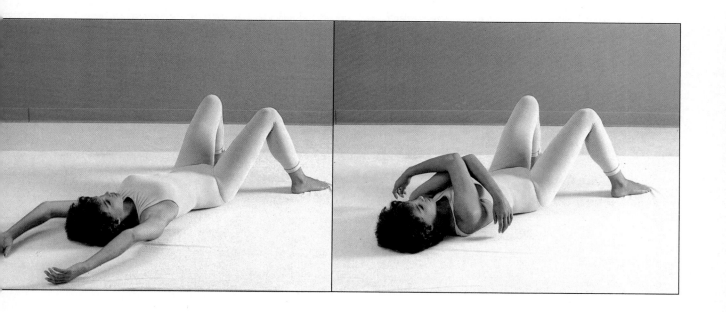

## Roll Down

Stand with your feet about two feet apart and raise your arms as if you were greeting the sky *(below left)*. Release the muscles in your hips, unlock your knees and slowly drop forward from the waist until your arms touch the floor. Roll back up to the start.

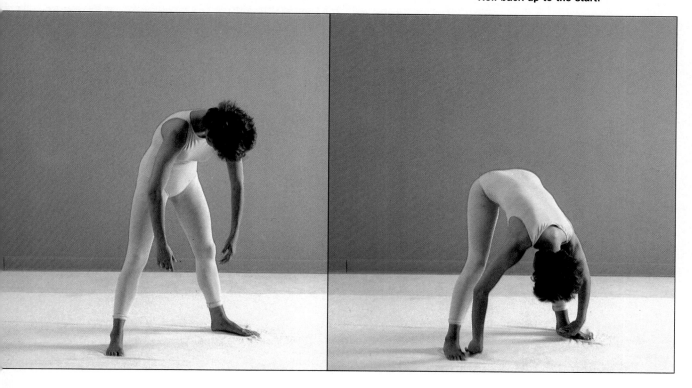

# Single-Arm Circle

Lie on the floor with your knees bent and your arms outstretched *(top)*. Drop your knees to the right and circle your left arm over your head as you roll onto your right side. Continue circling your left arm downward past your right arm *(bottom)* and, following the movement with your eyes, bring the left arm over your hip and back to its original position.

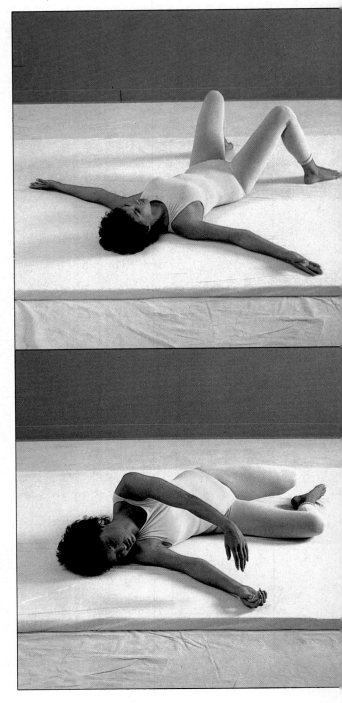

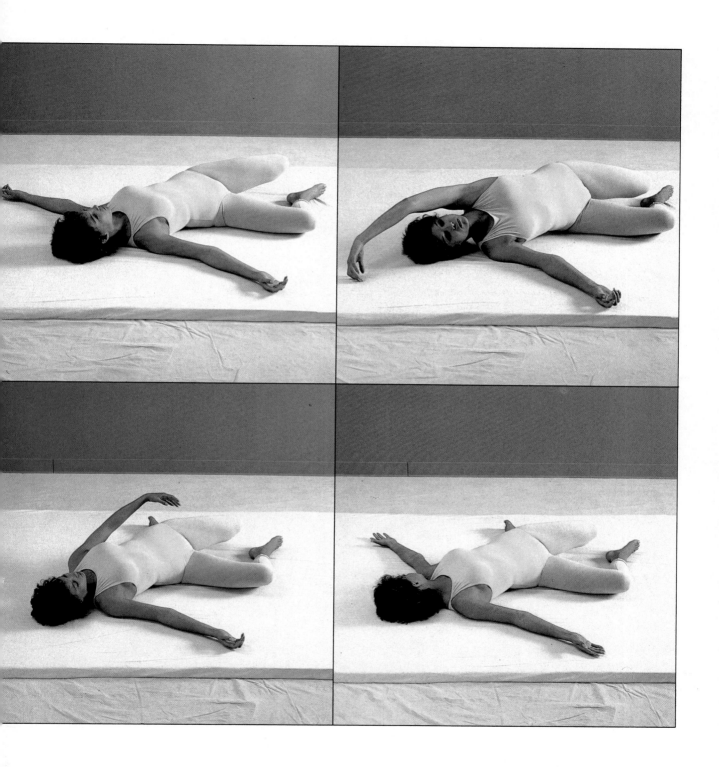

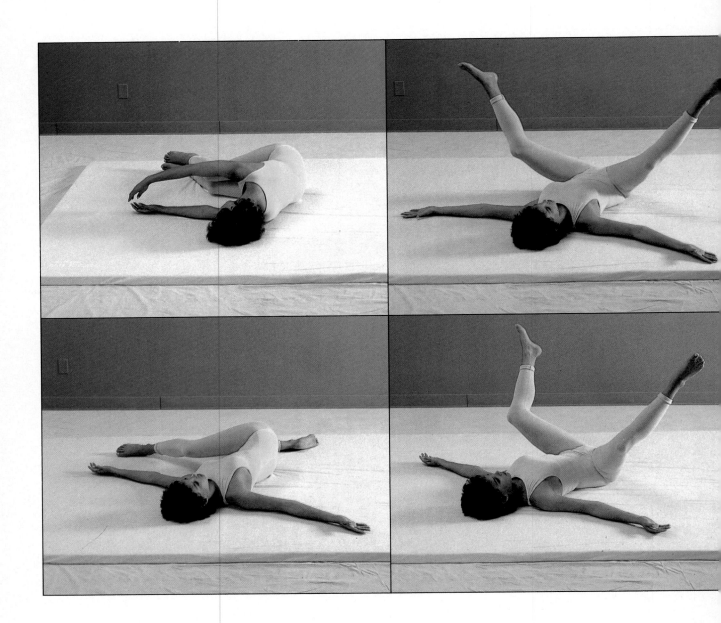

# Side-to-Side Roll

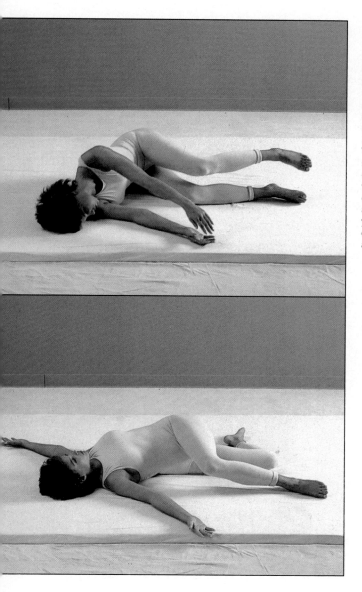

Lie on your side with your arms stretched parallel in front of you and your legs together, extending your feet but keeping your knees bent *(top)*. Slowly roll onto your back by opening your right arm and leg toward the right. Be sure to avoid arching your back. Continue rolling until you are resting on your other side. You can add a variation *(bottom)* by starting out lying with your arms outstretched and your hips and legs turned to the left. Keep your upper body open on the floor as you open your legs and roll them to the right. Be sure that your knees remain slightly bent and close enough to your torso so that you avoid arching your back.

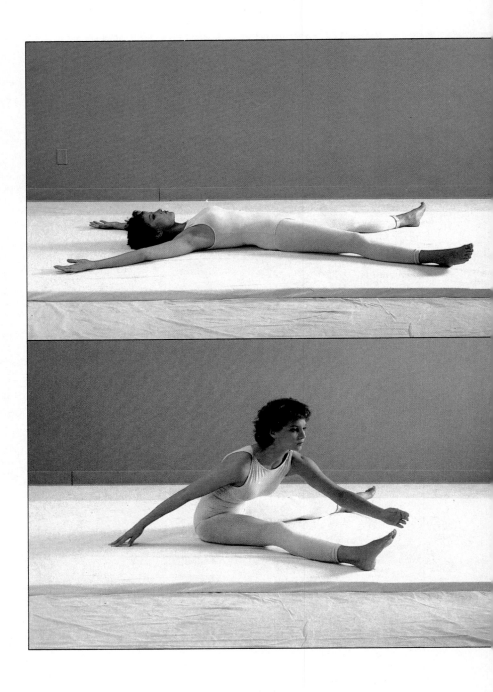

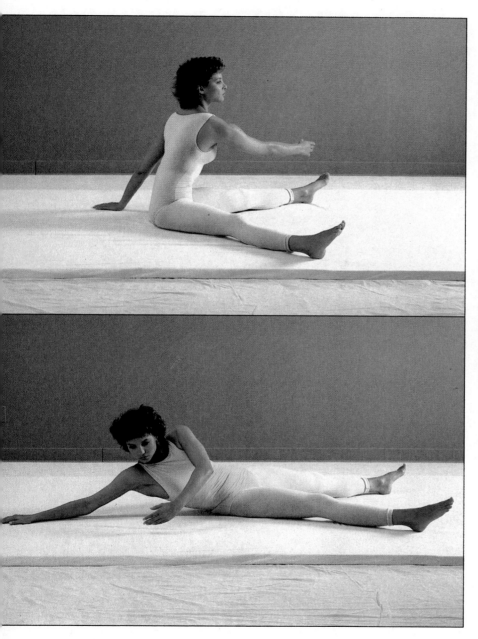

# Cross Reach

Lie flat on your back with your arms and legs extended and open *(top)*. Slide up on your left arm and reach with your right hand toward your left foot. Be sure not to lock your knees but keep them relaxed and bent slightly. Bend from the hips toward your foot without arching your back. Shift your support to your right arm and swing the left arm to your right foot *(bottom)*. Continue the swinging motion of your arm over your head and slide back down to the starting position.

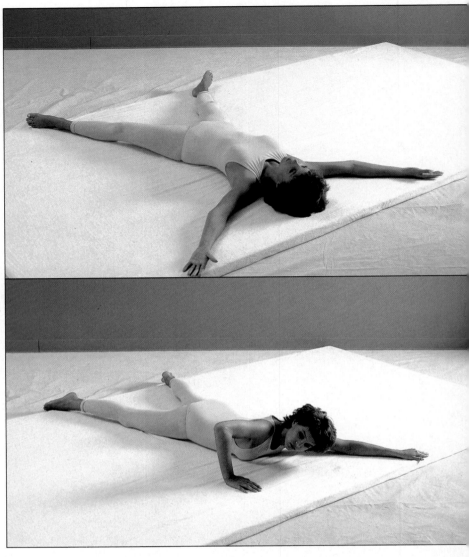

## Cross Roll

Lie flat on your back with your arms and legs extended wide to form an X *(top)*. Reach your left arm diagonally forward to the right and sit up. Twist to your right and support yourself with your right hand, sliding your left arm along the floor. Then bend your right elbow and drop your chest down, untwisting your legs *(middle)*. Reach your right arm away from the floor to roll over onto your back, with your upper body open but your torso and legs still twisted to the left. Finally, untwist your torso, drawing your right knee across your body and up *(bottom)*. Return to the starting position.

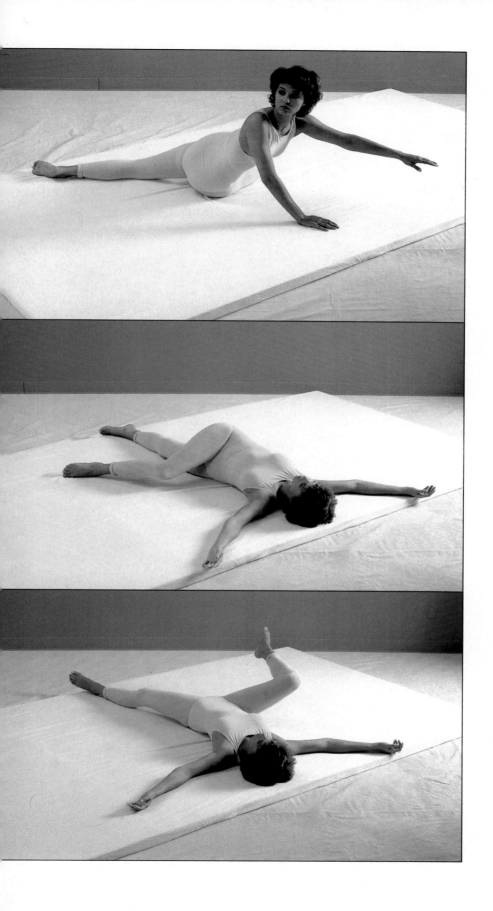

## Diagonal Reach

Standing with your feet apart, reach down with your right hand toward your left foot *(right)*. Be sure that your right leg is straight and your left knee is bent. Your back should feel stretched. Then open your chest by drawing your right hand up, leading with your elbow, until your arm is fully extended.

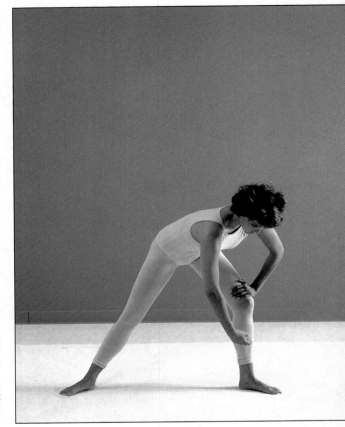

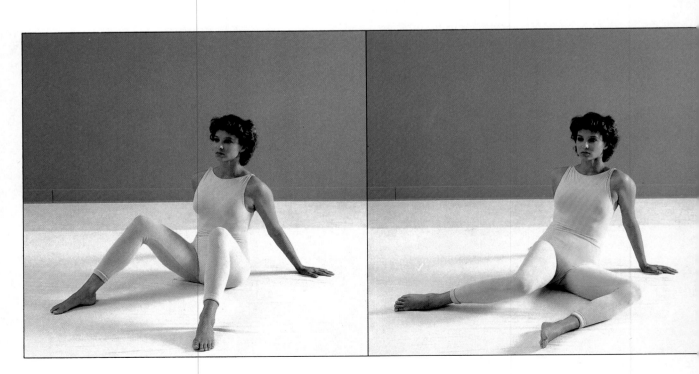

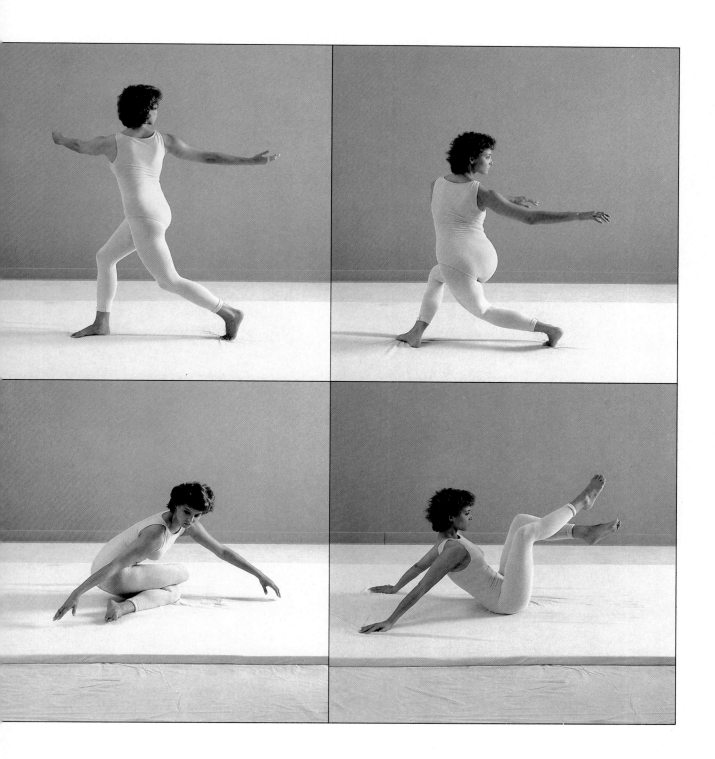

115

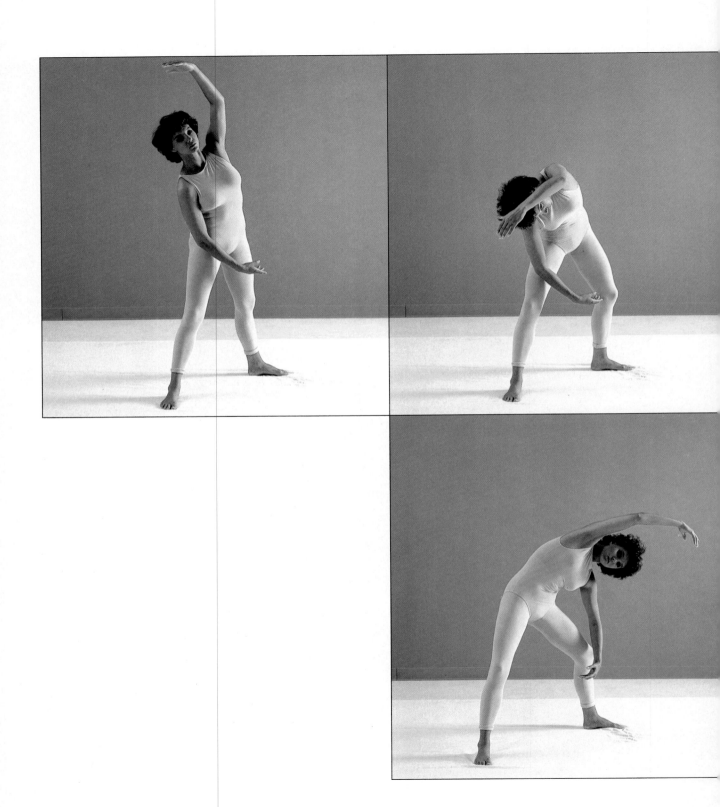

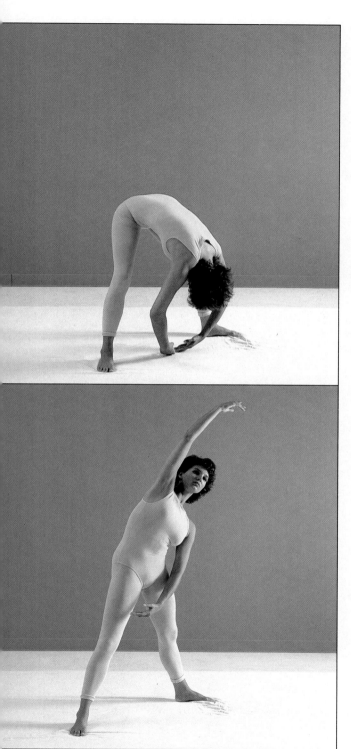

# Full-Body Circle

Standing with your feet apart, reach up with your left arm, stretching your left side *(top)*. Continue your arm reach in a circular motion, bending your knees slightly so that you can roll in a circle from the hips. Continue moving your right arm upward *(bottom)* and follow it with your body. As you return to an erect position, be sure you feel the extension through the waist, not the elbow.

# Salute to
# the Sun

This sequence, derived from a Yoga routine, uses almost every body part. Standing with arms outstretched, slowly bring your hands to the floor, bending your knees slightly *(top)*. Using your hands for support, extend one leg and then the other behind you, finally curling into a tucked position. Bring yourself out of the tuck *(bottom)* by drawing your chest forward and extending your body forward and up. Lift your hips and push yourself onto your feet, swinging your arms backward.

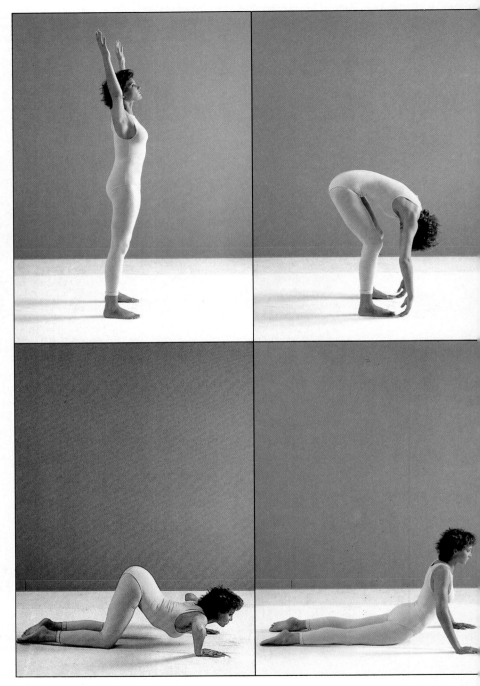

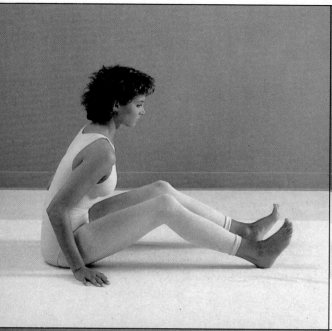

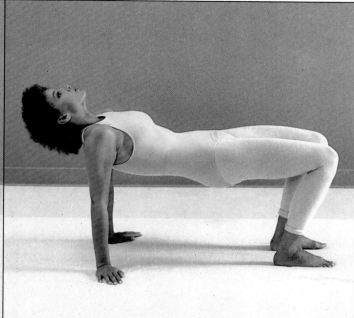

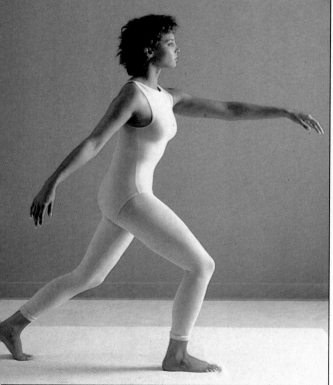

# Propulsion Sequence/2

You can add this sequence at the end of Propulsion Sequence/1 on pages 120-121, or you can use it as an exercise on its own. Start by sitting on your heels *(top)*. Walk your knees forward and come up on the balls of your feet. Then swing your hips backward and sit on the floor. Shift your lower body forward again, with your hips off your heels. Push forward onto your knees and bring your hands beneath you to the floor, extending one leg backward and the opposite hand forward *(bottom)*. Rise to a standing position, using your arms for balance and to achieve a smooth upward lift.

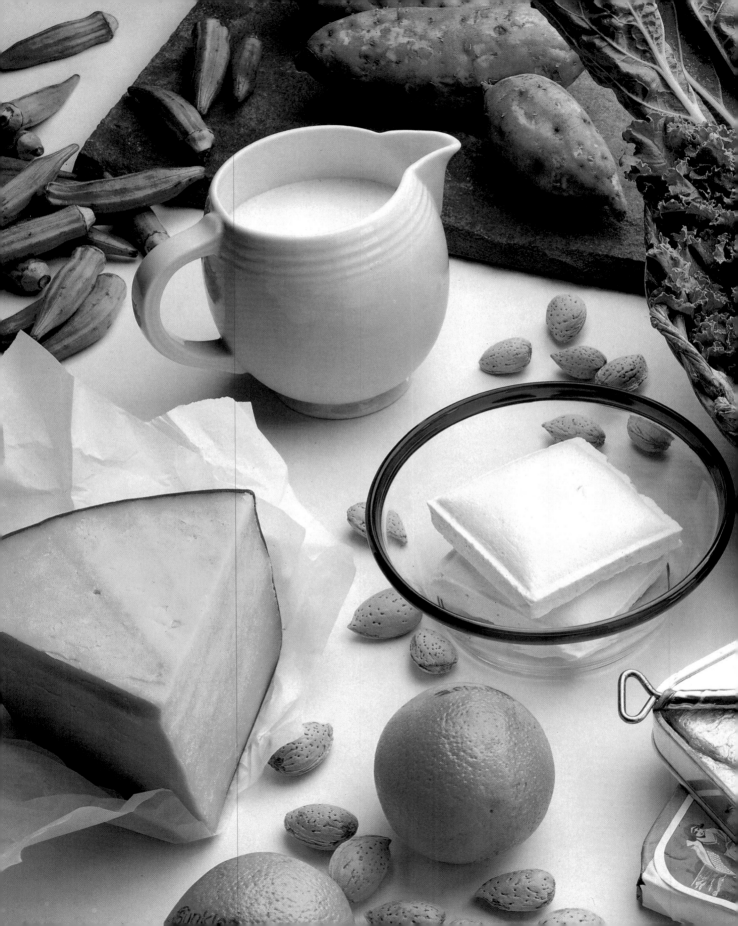

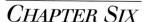

# CHAPTER SIX

# Calcium and Iron

*For flexible muscles, healthy bones and optimum energy — recipes with the right amounts of these minerals*

Four percent of your body weight consists of minerals. These inorganic substances help form your skeletal structure, keep your heart beating properly and supply your muscles with oxygen. Although there are more than 60 different minerals in the human body, scientists have identified only 20 as essential. Of these, calcium and iron are two of the most important.

Calcium is critical to the flexibility and operation of your muscles. An inadequate supply can result in muscle tightness and cramps. Calcium also maintains the flexibility of the spinal column. Without enough calcium, the weight-bearing vertebrae gradually compress, reducing your range of motion. And calcium combines with phosphorus to form and preserve your bones and teeth.

If you consistently fail to get enough calcium, you increase your risk of osteoporosis — porous bones. Your bones will become weak because your body has robbed a great deal of its skeletal calcium to get what it needs for vital everyday functions.

A major factor behind osteoporosis is a long-term calcium deficiency that begins in the early 20s, usually because of a lack of dairy products in the diet. Some researchers suspect that a lack of exercise also contributes to the onset of the disease, which is characterized by slow, progressive bone loss. Because of hormonal differences, women suffer from osteoporosis more frequently and at an earlier age than men. But now that their average life span exceeds 70 years, osteoporosis has become increasingly evident among older men as well.

Two of the first signs of osteoporosis are loss of height and reduced flexibility in your back. The disease takes a long time to manifest itself and usually is only detected when a bone fracture occurs. Though it may be slowed by increasing calcium intake, osteoporosis cannot be halted entirely, possibly because the body absorbs calcium much less efficiently after age 60; furthermore, less of the calcium you consume goes into your bones. To minimize bone loss, people over 60 should exercise regularly and should include sources of calcium in most of their meals. But to ensure healthy bones, you should begin consuming adequate amounts of calcium when you are young. This builds up a calcium reserve that will help compensate for your body's reduced ability to absorb calcium as you get older.

The generally recommended daily amount of calcium is 800 milligrams, the equivalent of about three 8-ounce glasses of milk. Unfortunately, one out of every four women gets less daily calcium than there is in one glass of milk. And half of all men over the age of 35 do not get the minimum requirement of calcium.

The best way to get calcium is in food. Vitamin D, which is present in or added to many calcium-filled dairy products, enhances your body's calcium absorption. When you use dairy products as a source of calcium, be sure to eat and drink lowfat or skim-milk products to keep your fat consumption down.

On average, three quarters of our dietary calcium comes from dairy products and the rest from plant foods. Besides dairy foods, other excellent animal sources of calcium are small fish, like sardines, that can be eaten with their soft bones intact. (The bones contain nearly all the calcium.) Tofu, molasses and leafy vegetables like collard greens are also good sources, though not as rich as animal sources.

Weight-bearing exercises such as running, walking, hiking and aerobic dancing increase calcium deposition in the bones of the lower body. A lack of this type of exercise slows calcium deposition, even when your dietary supply is adequate.

Your body contains much less iron than calcium: One sixth of an ounce of iron is the average as opposed to two to three pounds of calcium. But iron is just as important for good health. In the red blood cells, iron plays a key role in carrying oxygen to the muscles and other organs. Without enough iron, you will lose your appetite and feel sluggish. And, as is the case with calcium, iron deficiency often starts early in life when a person's diet excludes iron-rich foods.

Men normally need about 10 milligrams of iron daily, women about

# The Basic Guidelines

*For a moderately active adult, the National Institutes of Health recommends a diet that is low in fat, high in carbohydrates and moderate in protein. The institutes' guidelines suggest that no more than 30 percent of your calories come from fat, that 55 to 60 percent come from carbohydrates and that no more than 15 percent come from protein. A gram of fat equals nine calories, while a gram of protein or carbohydrate equals four calories; therefore, if you eat 2,100 calories a day, you should consume approximately 60 grams of fat, 315 grams of carbohydrate and no more than 75 grams of protein daily. If you follow a lowfat/high-carbohydrate diet, your chance of developing heart disease, cancer and other life-threatening diseases may be considerably reduced.*

◆ The nutrition charts that accompany each of the lowfat/high-carbohydrate recipes in this book include the number of calories per serving, the number of grams of fat, carbohydrate and protein in a serving, and the percentage of calories derived from each of these nutrients. In addition, the charts provide the amount of calcium, iron and sodium per serving.

◆ Calcium deficiency may be associated with periodontal disease — which attacks the mouth's bones and tissues, including the gums — in both men and women, and with osteoporosis, or bone shrinking and weakening, in the elderly. The deficiency may also contribute to high blood pressure. The recommended daily allowance for calcium is 800 milligrams a day for men and women. Pregnant and lactating women are advised to consume 1,200 milligrams daily; a National Institutes of Health consensus panel recommends that postmenopausal women consume 1,200 to 1,500 milligrams of calcium daily.

◆ Although one way you can reduce your fat intake is to cut your consumption of red meat, you should make sure that you get your necessary iron from other sources. The Food and Nutrition Board of the National Academy of Sciences suggests a minimum of 10 milligrams of iron per day for men and 18 milligrams for women between the ages of 11 and 50.

◆ High sodium intake is associated with high blood pressure. Most adults should restrict sodium intake to between 2,000 and 2,500 milligrams a day, according to the National Academy of Sciences. One way to keep sodium consumption in check is not to add table salt to food.

18 (because of blood loss during menstruation). The richest sources of iron are red meats, liver and egg yolks, but these also contain substantial amounts of fat and cholesterol. Good vegetarian sources are tofu, beans and iron-enriched cereals. These plant foods do not contain as much absorbable iron as animal products, but accompanying them with a small amount of meat or with foods high in vitamin C like tomatoes or citrus fruits enhances iron absorption. Strict vegetarians, though, may well need supplemental iron during early childhood, adolescence and pregnancy. (You should take supplements only after consulting a physician, since excessive iron intake can be toxic.)

It is a common belief that the only way to get adequate calcium and iron in your diet is by consuming relatively large quantities of milk and meat. In fact, this is not only unnecessary but unhealthy. The following recipes show how to draw on a healthy variety of sources to provide these two essential minerals.

# Breakfast

### HERBED MELON WITH YOGURT SAUCE

*Studies of soccer players, cross-country runners and other athletes show that weight-bearing exercise strengthens the bones of the lower body. This breakfast of melon and yogurt provides plenty of calcium, another way to help keep your bones strong.*

2 tablespoons honey
1 1/2 tablespoons lemon juice
1/4 cup minced fresh basil
2 tablespoons minced fresh mint

1/2 teaspoon coarsely ground black pepper
1 medium-size cantaloupe
1 cup plain lowfat yogurt

Combine 1 tablespoon of honey, the lemon juice, 1 1/2 tablespoons of basil, 1/2 tablespoon of mint and 1/4 teaspoon of pepper in a large bowl. Cut the cantaloupe into 1 1/2-inch cubes, add it to the bowl and toss to coat; set aside. Combine the yogurt, the remaining honey, herbs and pepper in a small bowl and stir well. Let the sauce stand for 15 minutes to allow the flavors to blend. Divide the cantaloupe and sauce between 2 large shallow bowls.

Makes 2 servings

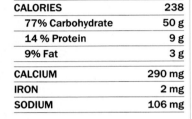

| CALORIES | 238 |
|---|---|
| 77% Carbohydrate | 50 g |
| 14 % Protein | 9 g |
| 9% Fat | 3 g |
| CALCIUM | 290 mg |
| IRON | 2 mg |
| SODIUM | 106 mg |

*Sweet Potato Slices with Canadian Bacon*

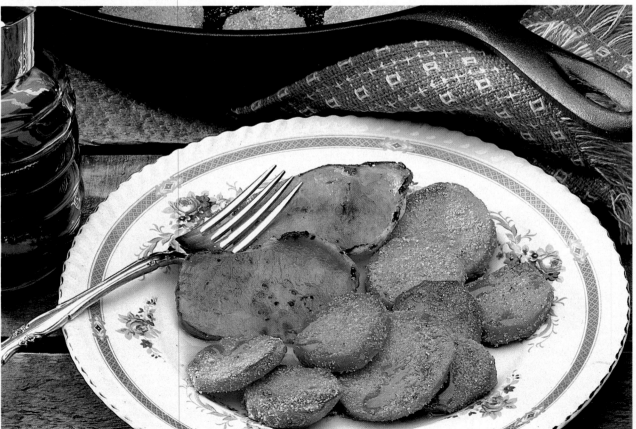

## CORIANDER AND CURRANT SCONES

*You can add calcium to your diet in cooked foods like these scones. The buttermilk they contain is an excellent lowfat calcium source.*

| | |
|---|---|
| 1 cup whole-wheat pastry flour | 3 tablespoons unsalted butter, well chilled |
| 1 cup unbleached all-purpose flour | |
| 1 tablespoon baking powder | 3/4 cup currants or raisins |
| 2 1/2 teaspoons ground coriander | 1 tablespoon grated orange peel |
| 1/2 teaspoon salt | 3/4 cup buttermilk |
| 1/2 teaspoon sugar | Vegetable cooking spray |

Combine the dry ingredients in a medium-size bowl. With a pastry blender or 2 knives, cut in the butter until the mixture resembles coarse meal. Scatter in the currants and orange peel, then with a fork stir in the buttermilk until just combined. Turn the dough out onto a floured board and knead it with floured hands 3 or 4 times. Spray a baking sheet with cooking spray. Divide the dough into 4 equal portions and shape each into a ball. Place the balls of dough on the baking sheet. With a sharp knife cut a cross in the top of each, then refrigerate for 15 minutes. Meanwhile, preheat the oven to 425° F. Bake the scones about 15 minutes, or until golden brown.          Makes 4 scones

Variation: For Shortcake Biscuits, omit the whole-wheat flour and use 2 cups of unbleached flour; omit the coriander, orange peel and currants. Roll the dough out 1 1/4 inches thick on a floured board and cut with a 3 1/2-inch round or heart-shaped cookie cutter. Bake as directed above. Use the biscuits for Fig-Berry Shortcakes (see page 137) and other desserts.

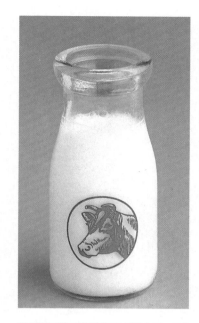

| CALORIES per scone | 398 |
|---|---|
| 70% Carbohydrate | 71 g |
| 8% Protein | 8 g |
| 22% Fat | 10 g |
| CALCIUM | 255 mg |
| IRON | 3 mg |
| SODIUM | 733 mg |

## SWEET POTATO SLICES WITH CANADIAN BACON

*Iron-rich molasses is the only sweetener that provides significant nutrients. According to Edward R. Eichner, M.D., a fellow of the American College of Sports Medicine, you can improve your iron absorption by not drinking coffee or tea (which inhibit iron uptake) with your meals.*

| | |
|---|---|
| 2 tablespoons maple syrup | 1 large sweet potato (about 1/2 pound), boiled and peeled |
| 1 tablespoon dark molasses | |
| 1/4 cup yellow cornmeal | 1 tablespoon unsalted butter |
| 3/4 teaspoon sugar | 2 thin slices Canadian bacon |
| 1/8 teaspoon salt | |

In a small bowl, stir together the maple syrup and molasses. Combine the cornmeal, sugar and salt in a shallow plate. Slice the potato into 1/4-inch-thick rounds and dredge in the cornmeal mixture until completely coated. Melt 1 1/2 teaspoons of butter in a large, heavy nonstick skillet over medium-high heat. Place a single layer of potato slices in the skillet and cook about 5 minutes, or until the undersides are lightly browned. Turn the potatoes, add the remaining butter to the skillet and cook another 5 minutes, or until lightly browned. Transfer the potatoes to a plate and wipe the skillet with paper towels. Add the bacon to the skillet and sear it over medium-high heat about 1 minute on each side, or until browned. Transfer the bacon to the plate with the potatoes and serve with the maple-molasses syrup.          Makes 1 serving

| CALORIES | 557 |
|---|---|
| 70% Carbohydrate | 99 g |
| 7% Protein | 10 g |
| 23% Fat | 14 g |
| CALCIUM | 230 mg |
| IRON | 6 mg |
| SODIUM | 726 mg |

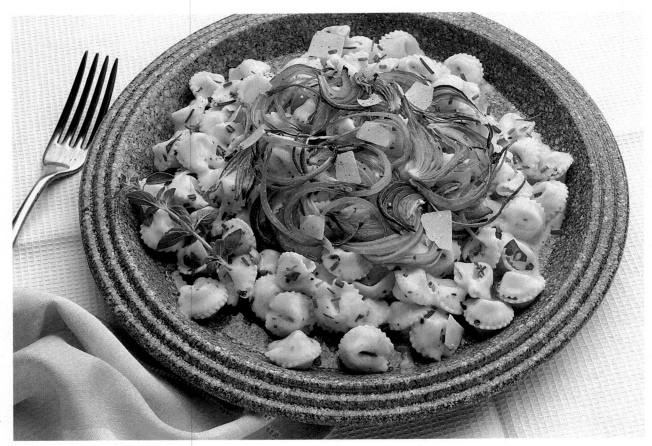

*Pasta with Goat Cheese and Onions*

# Lunch

### PASTA WITH GOAT CHEESE AND ONIONS

*Fortified skim milk contains vitamin D, a nutrient that aids calcium absorption. Although your skin produces vitamin D when exposed to sunlight, studies at the Tufts-USDA Nutrition Research Center show that the skin's ability to manufacture vitamin D decreases with age.*

| | |
|---|---|
| 6 ounces mild French goat cheese, such as Bucheron | Black pepper |
| 1/2 cup skim milk | 1/4 cup minced fresh herbs in any combination, such as basil, |
| 1 medium-size red onion | chives, Italian parsley, cilantro, |
| 1/2 teaspoon olive oil | thyme or rosemary |
| 1/2 pound capelletti or small shell pasta | 1 1/2 teaspoons Parmesan, shaved or grated |

| CALORIES | 471 |
|---|---|
| 54% Carbohydrate | 63 g |
| 18% Protein | 21 g |
| 28% Fat | 15 g |
| CALCIUM | 334 mg |
| IRON | 3 mg |
| SODIUM | 580 mg |

Bring enough water to a boil in the bottom of a double boiler so that the boiling water will just touch the top pan. When the water boils, place the cheese in the top pan and heat, stirring with a whisk, until the cheese is completely melted. Whisk in the skim milk, cover the pan and set aside.

Bring a large pot of water to a boil. Preheat the broiler and position the rack

130

2 inches from the heat. Slice the onion into 1/8-inch-thick wedges; do not separate the layers. Place a nonstick baking sheet under the broiler 1 minute, or until hot. Arrange the onion wedges in a single layer on the sheet and brush the tops and sides of the slices lightly with oil. Broil the onions about 5 minutes, or until they are soft and slightly charred.

Cook the pasta in the boiling water until al dente, drain well and return to the pot. Add the cheese mixture, black pepper to taste and half the fresh herbs and toss well. Divide the pasta among 3 dinner plates and top with equal amounts of charred onions and Parmesan. Sprinkle with the remaining herbs and serve.

*Makes 3 servings*

## VEGETABLE-CHEESE BURRITOS

*Spinach and other dark leafy greens are high in iron, fiber, potassium, vitamin A and vitamin C.*

2 packed cups arugula, watercress or spinach leaves, coarsely chopped

1 large tomato, cored and cut into 1-inch pieces

3/4 cup crumbled feta cheese

1 tablespoon minced red onion

1 red bell pepper, roasted, peeled and finely diced

1 garlic clove, minced

1 tablespoon red wine vinegar, preferably balsamic

1 1/2 teaspoons dried oregano

Six 8-inch flour tortillas

| CALORIES | 299 |
|---|---|
| 57% Carbohydrate | 43 g |
| 14% Protein | 11 g |
| 29% Fat | 10 g |
| CALCIUM | 274 mg |
| IRON | 4 mg |
| SODIUM | 331 mg |

Combine the chopped greens, tomato, feta, onion, bell pepper, garlic and vinegar in a large bowl. Heat a large skillet over high heat. Sprinkle 1/4 teaspoon of oregano over the surface of the skillet. When the oregano is just smoking, add one tortilla and heat for about 30 seconds. Remove the tortilla from the skillet and place one sixth of the vegetable mixture in the center. Fold the bottom third of the tortilla over the filling, then roll the sides together loosely. Repeat with the remaining tortillas and filling, and serve.

*Makes 3 servings*

## CHILLED MANGO SOUP

*Nancy Clark, one of the country's foremost sports nutritionists, recommends a milk-based soup like this one to add extra calcium to a meal.*

1 ripe mango (1 pound, or about 1 1/3 cups pulp)

2 cups buttermilk

4 tablespoons nonfat dry milk

1/4 cup lime juice

1 cup seltzer

1 large cucumber, seeded and finely diced

1 small fresh hot red pepper, chopped

4 teaspoons minced fresh cilantro, basil or mint

| CALORIES | 133 |
|---|---|
| 72% Carbohydrate | 26 g |
| 19% Protein | 7 g |
| 9% Fat | 1 g |
| CALCIUM | 220 mg |
| IRON | .6 mg |
| SODIUM | 156 mg |

Halve and pit the mango and scoop the flesh into the container of a blender. Add the buttermilk, nonfat dry milk and lime juice, and purée until smooth. (This mixture can be made in advance and refrigerated until serving time.) Just before serving, stir in the seltzer and divide the soup among 4 bowls. Divide the cucumber equally among the bowls and sprinkle each serving with red pepper and herbs.

*Makes 4 servings*

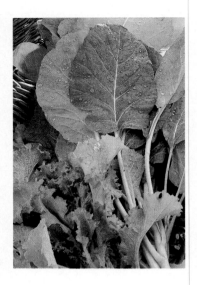

| CALORIES | 202 |
|---|---|
| 29% Carbohydrate | 16 g |
| 29% Protein | 16 g |
| 42% Fat | 10 g |
| CALCIUM | 308 mg |
| IRON | 4 mg |
| SODIUM | 295 mg |

## FRITTATA WITH GREENS AND TOFU

*This quick lunch or dinner dish gets its iron boost from tofu and greens, and is an excellent source of protein and calcium as well.*

1 pound trimmed mustard,
 turnip or collard greens,
 coarsely chopped, or 10-ounce
 package frozen greens, thawed
1 1/2 teaspoons olive oil
1/2 cup coarsely chopped shallots
6 garlic cloves, minced
2 whole anchovies, bone in,
 rinsed, dried and finely chopped

1/4 teaspoon red pepper flakes
1 teaspoon dried thyme
6 ounces firm tofu, cut into 1/4-inch
 cubes
3 large eggs
3 tablespoons skim milk
1/4 teaspoon salt
1 1/2 ounces part skim-milk
 mozzarella, cut into thin strips

If using fresh greens, place in a large nonstick skillet with 1/2 cup water, cover and cook over medium-low heat about 20 minutes, or until tender. Uncover the skillet and cook until the moisture evaporates. Transfer the greens to a large bowl; you should have about 2 cups. If using frozen greens, drain and squeeze enough dry to measure 2 cups; set aside.

Heat the oil in a large nonstick skillet over medium heat. Add the shallots, garlic, anchovies, red pepper flakes and thyme, and cook about 10 minutes, or until the shallots and garlic are softened. Add the greens and tofu to the skillet, toss to coat well and distribute the mixture evenly in the skillet.

In a medium-size bowl beat together the eggs, milk and salt and pour the mixture into the skillet, pressing the egg mixture evenly into the greens and tofu with a wooden spoon. Cook, covered, over medium heat for 3 to 4 minutes, or until the eggs are set. Lay the mozzarella strips on top of the frittata, reduce the heat to low, cover and cook about 1 minute, or just until the cheese melts. Serve hot or warm. Makes 4 servings

## HEARTY SQUASH SOUP

*The acorn squash used in this thick, rich soup is a good source of iron and provides a substantial amount of vitamin A and protein.*

2 acorn squashes (1 1/2
 pounds each)
1/4 cup low-sodium chicken stock
4 large shallots, minced
1 teaspoon olive oil
2 tablespoons dry white wine
3/4 cup evaporated skimmed milk
3/4 teaspoon black pepper

1/4 teaspoon salt
Four 1/4-inch-thick slices
 whole-wheat Italian bread
2/3 cup grated part skim-milk
 mozzarella
1/2 cup grated Gruyère cheese
2 tablespoons minced fresh basil

| CALORIES | 639 |
|---|---|
| 57% Carbohydrate | 95 g |
| 19% Protein | 33 g |
| 24% Fat | 18 g |
| CALCIUM | 985 mg |
| IRON | 6 mg |
| SODIUM | 878 mg |

Preheat the oven to 400° F. Cut off a 1 1/2-inch-thick "lid" from the stem end of each squash. Cut a thin slice off the bottom of each squash, then scoop out and discard the seeds and stringy membranes. Place the squashes upright and the lids cut side up on a foil-lined baking sheet. Place 2 tablespoons of stock in each squash and cover loosely with foil. Bake 40 minutes, or until the squashes are just tender but still hold their shape.

Meanwhile, in a small saucepan over medium heat sauté the shallots in the oil until they just begin to brown. Add the wine and cook, stirring, until it evaporates. Remove the pan from the heat. When the squashes are cooked, carefully scoop out the flesh with a teaspoon, leaving a 1/2-inch-thick shell and being careful not to pierce the skin. Add the scooped-out flesh, the milk, pepper and salt to the shallots and cook over medium heat until hot, mashing the squash with a wooden spoon. Spoon one sixth of the mixture into each hollowed-out squash and top with a slice of bread. Sprinkle with one sixth of the cheese and top with another one sixth of the squash mixture. Repeat the layers of bread, squash and cheese until the squashes are filled, finishing with a layer of cheese. Return the lids and squashes to the oven and bake for 10 minutes, or until the cheese is melted. Sprinkle each serving with basil, cover the squashes with the lids and serve.

Makes 2 servings

## SARDINE CAKES WITH TARRAGON-MUSTARD SAUCE

*Always eat sardines with the bones, which are the source of calcium.*

2 leeks
1 tablespoon olive oil
Two 3 3/4-ounce cans low-sodium, water-packed sardines
2 medium-size baking potatoes (about 1 pound), boiled in their skins, peeled and mashed

1 large egg
1/4 teaspoon dried thyme
1/8 teaspoon black pepper
1 teaspoon grated lemon peel
1/4 teaspoon anchovy paste
Tarragon-Mustard Sauce (recipe follows)

Trim the leeks, discarding the green leaves. Split and carefully wash the leeks and slice them thinly; you should have about 1 cup. Heat the oil in a small skillet over medium-high heat, add the leeks and cook about 6 minutes, or until softened. Add 1 tablespoon of water to prevent sticking, if necessary. Set aside to cool. Reserving 1/2 can for another use, drain and pat dry 1 1/2 cans of sardines and crumble them into a large bowl. Add the leeks, potatoes, egg, thyme, pepper, lemon peel and anchovy paste, and stir to combine. Heat a large nonstick skillet over medium-high heat. Form 1/4-cup portions of the sardine mixture into 12 patties and cook about 2 minutes on each side, or until browned. Serve with Tarragon-Mustard Sauce.

Makes 6 servings

| CALORIES without sauce | 165 |
| --- | --- |
| 41% Carbohydrate | 17 g |
| 17% Protein | 7 g |
| 42% Fat | 8 g |
| CALCIUM | 99 mg |
| IRON | 1 mg |
| SODIUM | 51 mg |

## TARRAGON-MUSTARD SAUCE

1 teaspoon dry mustard
1/4 cup dill pickle juice
2 teaspoons dried tarragon
1/2 cup nonbutterfat sour dressing

4 teaspoons minced shallot
2 teaspoons minced fresh parsley
1/4 cup minced dill pickle
1/2 teaspoon minced garlic
1/8 teaspoon sugar

In a medium-size bowl dissolve the mustard in the pickle juice. Add the tarragon and set aside for 5 minutes. Add the sour dressing, shallot, parsley, pickle, garlic and sugar, and stir to combine.

Makes 1 cup

Note: Nonbutterfat sour dressing is a lowfat sour cream substitute available at most supermarkets.

| CALORIES per tablespoon | 13 |
| --- | --- |
| 25% Carbohydrate | 1 g |
| 8% Protein | .4 g |
| 67% Fat | 1 g |
| CALCIUM | 5 mg |
| IRON | .1 mg |
| SODIUM | 166 mg |

# Dinner

## LIVER AND FIGS EN BROCHETTE

*Although liver is an outstanding source of iron, protein and B vitamins, it also contains a fair amount of saturated fat and cholesterol. You should not eat it more than twice a week.*

| CALORIES | 553 |
|---|---|
| 58% Carbohydrate | 84 g |
| 18% Protein | 25 g |
| 24% Fat | 16 g |
| CALCIUM | 239 mg |
| IRON | 13 mg |
| SODIUM | 593 mg |

2 red onions (about 1 1/4 pounds)
1 tablespoon dry sherry
2 2/3 tablespoons olive oil
1 teaspoon dried thyme, crushed
1/2 teaspoon dried sage, crumbled
1/2 teaspoon coarsely ground black pepper
4 garlic cloves, minced

3/8 teaspoon salt
24 large whole bay leaves
3/4 pound calf's liver, cut into sixteen 1-inch cubes
1/2 pound dried figs (6 to 10 figs), halved
1 baguette (long, slender loaf of bread), preferably sourdough

Leaving the root end intact, cut each onion lengthwise into six to eight 1-inch-wide wedges. In a medium-size bowl combine the sherry, 1 tablespoon of olive oil, the thyme, sage, pepper, garlic and 1/4 teaspoon of salt. Add the onions, bay leaves, liver and figs and toss to coat with the marinade. Cover and marinate in the refrigerator for 3 to 4 hours or overnight.

Preheat the broiler and position the rack 4 inches from the heat. Alternately thread 4 liver cubes, 6 bay leaves and 4 or 5 fig halves onto each of four 8- to 10-inch skewers. Lay the onion wedges on a baking sheet, brush with 1

*Liver and Figs en Brochette*

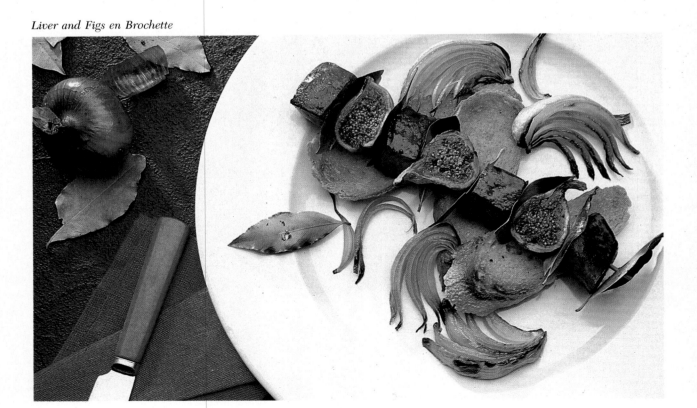

teaspoon of oil and sprinkle with 1/8 teaspoon of salt. Cut the baguette on the diagonal into twelve 1/2-inch-thick slices and brush with the remaining oil; set aside. Broil the onions, turning halfway through cooking, about 7 minutes, or until they are soft and slightly blackened at the ends. Divide the onions among 4 plates. Place the bread slices on the baking sheet and broil them about 1 1/2 minutes, or until lightly browned on top. Transfer the bread to the plates. Place the liver on a broiler pan and broil, turning halfway through cooking, about 6 minutes, or until the liver looks browned. Do not worry if the bay leaves smoke a bit. Transfer the skewers to the plates and serve. Note: The bay leaves are for flavoring only and should not be eaten.

Makes 4 servings

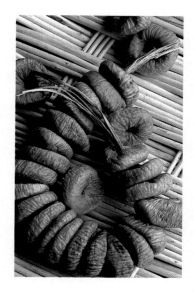

## LINGUINE WITH FIGS AND WALNUTS

*This dish would be good to include in a recovery meal following an endurance event. The cheese is an excellent source of protein and calcium, and the figs supply potassium, an important mineral lost in perspiration.*

2 tablespoons olive oil, preferably extra-virgin

7 garlic cloves, peeled and thinly sliced

2 anchovy fillets, rinsed, dried and finely chopped

3 leeks, white part only, thinly sliced

10 dried figs, cut into 1/2 x 1/8-inch pieces

1 tablespoon dry white wine

5 tablespoons low-sodium chicken stock

1/4 cup coarsely chopped walnuts

1/4 cup minced Italian parsley

1/2 pound linguine

1/4 teaspoon salt

Black pepper

1 1/2 ounces Parmesan, shaved or grated

| CALORIES | 696 |
|---|---|
| 62% Carbohydrate | 109g |
| 11% Protein | 21 g |
| 27% Fat | 22 g |
| CALCIUM | 374 mg |
| IRON | 6 mg |
| SODIUM | 571 mg |

Bring a large pot of water to a boil. Meanwhile, for the sauce, heat 1 tablespoon of the oil in a medium-size nonstick skillet over medium heat. Add the garlic and sauté about 5 minutes, or until the garlic just begins to brown. Stir in the anchovy fillets, then add the leeks and figs. Cover the skillet, reduce the heat slightly and cook about 8 minutes, or until the leeks are tender. Stir in the wine and cook for 45 seconds. Stir in the chicken stock, walnuts and half of the parsley and cook for another minute. Remove the skillet from the heat, cover to keep warm and set aside.

   Cook the linguine in the boiling water until al dente, drain and return to the pot. Add the remaining olive oil and parsley, the salt, and pepper to taste, and toss. Divide the linguine between 2 bowls and spoon an equal amount of sauce and Parmesan cheese over each. Serve immediately.

Makes 2 servings

## SEAFOOD AND BROCCOLI SALAD
## WITH BLACK BEAN DRESSING

*Scallops are high in protein and iron, and also lower in cholesterol than most seafood. Steaming vegetables rather than boiling them preserves the maximum amount of nutrients.*

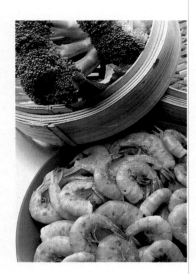

1 tablespoon safflower oil
2 tablespoons chopped fresh
  ginger
1 1/2 tablespoons chopped garlic
4 tablespoons chopped scallions
1/4 teaspoon red pepper flakes
1 tablespoon Chinese salted black
  beans, rinsed
2 teaspoons reduced-sodium soy
  sauce

2 teaspoons Japanese rice-wine
  vinegar
3/4 pound broccoli, cut into 1-inch
  florets, stems peeled and cut into
  1/2-inch pieces
1/4 pound medium-size shrimp
1/4 pound sea scallops
Small firm pear, such as a Bosc

For the dressing, heat the oil in a large skillet over medium-high heat. Add the ginger, garlic, scallions, pepper flakes and black beans, and cook for 5 to 6 minutes, or until the garlic is golden. Add the soy sauce, vinegar and 1 tablespoon of water, and cook for another 30 seconds. Transfer the mixture to a medium-size bowl and set aside.

Bring 1 inch of water to a boil in a covered saucepan large enough to hold a vegetable steamer. When the water boils, place the broccoli and shrimp in the steamer, cover, and cook about 4 minutes, or until the broccoli is bright green and the shrimp are pink and almost cooked. Add the scallops and steam for another minute. Transfer the broccoli and scallops to the bowl of dressing. Peel the shrimp, add to the broccoli and scallops, and toss well. Divide the salad between 2 plates, reserving some of the dressing. Halve, core and peel the pear and cut it into 1/4-inch dice. Toss the diced pear with the reserved dressing and place in the center of each serving of salad.

Makes 2 servings

Note: Chinese salted black beans (sometimes called fermented black beans) are soybeans that have been cooked, seasoned and then aged for several months. They are used in small amounts for flavoring. Salted black beans are sold in cans or plastic bags in Chinese food stores and will keep indefinitely in a tightly closed jar at room temperature. Japanese rice-wine vinegar is mild and slightly sweet. Substitute mild cider vinegar or white vinegar if rice-wine vinegar is unavailable.

| CALORIES | 267 |
|---|---|
| 38% Carbohydrate | 27 g |
| 36% Protein | 25 g |
| 26% Fat | 8 g |
| CALCIUM | 162 mg |
| IRON | 4 mg |
| SODIUM | 462 mg |

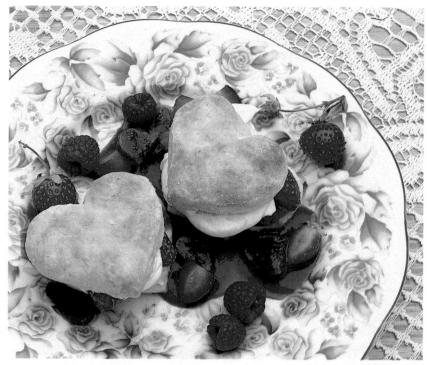

*Fig-Berry Shortcakes*

# Desserts

### FIG-BERRY SHORTCAKES

*Besides containing iron and calcium, figs are also extremely high in fiber.*
*Be sure to drink plenty of fluids with them to aid digestion.*

| CALORIES | 571 |
|---|---|
| 71% Carbohydrate | 105 g |
| 10% Protein | 15 g |
| 19% Fat | 13 g |
| CALCIUM | 336 mg |
| IRON | 4 mg |
| SODIUM | 769 mg |

10 dried figs
1/2 vanilla bean, split, seeds
    scraped out and reserved
2 cups each strawberries and
    raspberries
2 tablespoons honey

4 Shortcake Biscuits (see Coriander
    and Currant Scones recipe, page
    129)
1/2 cup Honey Cream (recipe
    follows)

For the fig-berry sauce, place the figs and the vanilla bean halves and seeds in a 1-quart saucepan, add water to cover and bring to a boil. Reduce the heat and simmer about 10 minutes, or until the figs are tender. Meanwhile, wash the berries and hull and slice the strawberries. Combine 1 cup each of the raspberries and strawberries with the honey in a food processor, and purée. Strain the purée into a medium-size bowl and set aside. When the figs are cooked, drain them and, when cool enough to handle, quarter them and cut into thin slices. Reserving a few berries for garnish, stir the remaining berries and the figs into the purée. Chill the mixture until ready to serve.

To serve, split the biscuits in half. Spoon one fourth of the fig-berry sauce onto the bottom of each biscuit, then top with 2 tablespoons of Honey Cream. Cover with the biscuit tops and garnish with whole berries if desired.

Makes 4 servings

137

| CALORIES per tablespoon | 20 |
| --- | --- |
| 26% Carbohydrate | 1 g |
| 37% Protein | 2 g |
| 37% Fat | .8 g |
| CALCIUM | 9 mg |
| IRON | .01 mg |
| SODIUM | 59 mg |

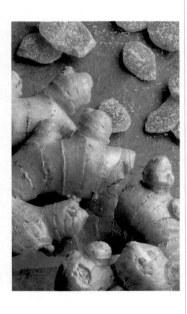

| CALORIES | 257 |
| --- | --- |
| 74% Carbohydrate | 48 g |
| 15% Protein | 10 g |
| 11% Fat | 3 g |
| CALCIUM | 181 mg |
| IRON | 4 mg |
| SODIUM | 210 mg |

# HONEY CREAM

*Use this lowfat alternative to whipped cream as a topping on fresh or cooked fruit to create desserts that are rich in calcium yet lower in fat. It can also replace butter and syrup on pancakes or waffles.*

1 cup no-salt-added lowfat cottage cheese (1% fat)
2 teaspoons honey

5 tablespoons nonbutterfat sour dressing

Purée the cottage cheese in a food processor or blender until smooth. Transfer the cheese to a small bowl and fold in the honey and sour dressing. Cover the bowl and refrigerate the mixture until ready to use. Honey Cream will keep for a week refrigerated in a covered container.                Makes 1 cup

# GINGER SOUFFLES

*This dish supplies complete protein as well as healthy amounts of vitamins and minerals. The sweet potatoes provide protein, vitamin A and potassium as well as vitamin C, which aids absorption of the iron from the molasses. The egg whites add extra protein without the cholesterol present in yolks. The nonfat dry milk and evaporated skimmed milk are packed with protein and calcium but contain virtually no fat.*

Vegetable cooking spray
2 medium-size sweet potatoes (about 3/4 pound total weight), boiled, peeled and cut into chunks
1/4 cup nonfat dry milk
2 tablespoons evaporated skimmed milk
1 1/2 ounces crystallized ginger, chopped

2 tablespoons grated fresh ginger
4 teaspoons molasses
1 tablespoon honey
1/2 teaspoon vanilla extract
2 eggs, separated, plus 4 egg whites
1/8 teaspoon cream of tartar
1/8 teaspoon salt
3 tablespoons sugar

Preheat the oven to 425° F. Spray four 12-ounce soufflé dishes with cooking spray. Place the dishes on a baking sheet and set aside. Purée the sweet potatoes in a food processor until perfectly smooth, then transfer the purée to a medium-size bowl. Whisk in the nonfat dry milk, evaporated skimmed milk, crystallized and fresh ginger, molasses, honey, vanilla and the 2 egg yolks. In another medium-size bowl, using an electric mixer beat the 6 egg whites, the cream of tartar and salt until soft peaks form. While continuing to beat, sprinkle in the sugar 1 tablespoon at a time and beat until stiff peaks form. Using a rubber spatula, fold 1/3 of the whites into the sweet potato mixture, then gently fold in the remaining whites until incorporated, being careful not to deflate the mixture. Divide the mixture among the prepared soufflé dishes, mounding slightly in the centers. Place the baking sheet with the soufflés in the oven and immediately reduce the temperature to 375° F. Bake the soufflés for 15 to 17 minutes, or until they are puffed and browned. Serve immediately.
Makes 4 servings

# FRESH FRUIT WITH WARM CUSTARD

*Iron from plant sources like raspberries is not as well absorbed by the body as the iron in animal foods. But, according to Ann C. Grandjean, nutrition advisor to the U.S. Olympic Committee, accompanying such iron sources with foods rich in vitamin C (such as the strawberries in this recipe) will enhance the amount of iron your body absorbs.*

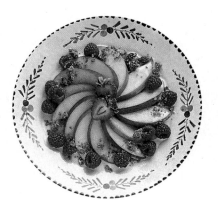

**2 cups evaporated skimmed milk**
**1/4 cup honey**
**Three 1 x 3-inch strips orange peel**
**1 1/2 teaspoons fennel seeds**
**1 vanilla bean, split, seeds**
**scraped out and reserved**
**3 egg yolks**

**2 cups each strawberries and**
**raspberries, or 4 cups of either**
**2 nectarines or peaches, thinly**
**sliced (2 cups)**
**4 amaretti (Italian almond cookies),**
**coarsely crushed**

For the custard, bring enough water to a boil in the bottom of a double boiler so that the boiling water will just touch the top pan. In the top pan combine the milk, honey, orange peel, fennel seeds and vanilla bean halves and seeds. Cook, covered, over the boiling water 15 minutes. Whisk in the egg yolks and cook, uncovered, stirring occasionally, about 15 minutes, or until the mixture coats the back of a wooden spoon. Reduce the heat and keep the custard warm until ready to serve.

Just before serving, wash and dry the berries and hull and slice the strawberries, if using. Mound half of the berries on 4 dessert plates and lay the nectarine slices pinwheel-fashion on top. Arrange the remaining berries decoratively on the plate. Strain the warm custard into a measuring cup; discard the vanilla bean and seeds. Pour 1/4 cup of custard over each serving, then sprinkle the fruit and custard with the crushed amaretti.         Makes 4 servings

Note: Amaretti are Italian almond macaroons made without egg yolks or shortening. They are sold in specialty food shops and the gourmet-food sections of some supermarkets. If amaretti are unavailable, substitute other plain cookies, such as gingersnaps or graham crackers.

| CALORIES | 333 |
|---|---|
| 67% Carbohydrate | 58 g |
| 16% Protein | 14 g |
| 17% Fat | 7 g |
| CALCIUM | 476 mg |
| IRON | 3 mg |
| SODIUM | 166 mg |

# Snacks and Beverages

### ANTIPASTO SNACK

*This mixture of pickled fruits and vegetables, a variation on an Italian condiment, makes a delicious snack or appetizer. The okra and dried fruits supply calcium, potassium and fiber, and the apricots, like most deep-yellow fruits and vegetables, are also rich in vitamin A.*

| CALORIES | | 399 |
|---|---|---|
| | 68% Carbohydrate | 71 g |
| | 13% Protein | 14 g |
| | 19% Fat | 9 g |
| CALCIUM | | 346 mg |
| IRON | | 4 mg |
| SODIUM | | 488 mg |

1 1/2 pounds fresh okra
3/4 pound pitted prunes (about 40)
1 pound yellow onions, peeled
   and thinly sliced
1/4 pound dried apricots (about 16)
1 sprig fresh thyme
1 medium-size fresh or dried hot
   red pepper

4 garlic cloves, peeled
4 cups white wine vinegar
2 tablespoons coriander seeds
2 tablespoons sugar
1/4 teaspoon coarse salt
4 bay leaves
1/2 pound provolone cheese
16 breadsticks

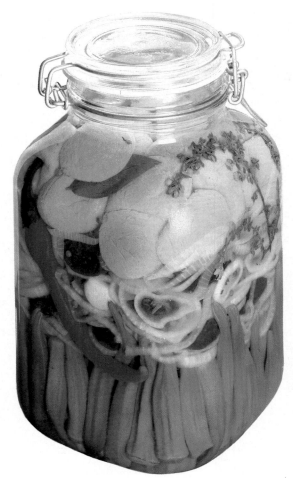

*Antipasto Snack*

Wash and trim the okra and pack the pods vertically into a 3-quart canning jar. Toss the prunes with the onion slices and place the mixture on top of the okra. Place the apricots on top of the prunes and onions and tuck the thyme sprig, red pepper and garlic cloves down into the jar. In a nonreactive saucepan combine 3 cups of water with the vinegar, coriander seeds, sugar, salt and bay leaves, and bring to a rolling boil. Pour the boiling liquid into the jar, filling it to the top. Let cool, then close the jar tightly and refrigerate for 2 to 3 days to allow the flavors to develop. Accompany each serving with 1 ounce of provolone and 2 breadsticks.

Makes 8 servings

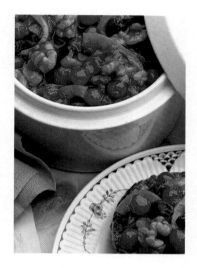

## CRANBERRY-WALNUT CONSERVE

*Spread this conserve on whole-wheat bread, or stir it into plain lowfat yogurt, to add calcium, protein, iron and fiber. It can also be served as a relish with poultry. A conserve is a chunky preserve made from several kinds of fruit.*

5 cups fresh or frozen cranberries

3 navel oranges, skins left on, quartered and thinly sliced

3/4 cup honey

1 1/4 cups dark raisins

1 1/2 cups coarsely chopped walnuts

1/4 cup lime or lemon juice, preferably freshly squeezed

In a heavy nonreactive 3-quart saucepan, combine 4 cups of cranberries, the oranges, honey and 1 1/2 cups of hot water, and bring to a boil over medium-high heat. Reduce the heat to medium and cook, stirring occasionally, about 15 minutes, or until the mixture has thickened and the cranberries are soft. Stir in the raisins and remaining cranberries and cook another 4 minutes, or until the raisins are plump. Remove the pan from the heat and stir in the walnuts and juice. Transfer the conserve to a glass or ceramic bowl, crock or jar, cover and chill before serving. The conserve keeps for up to a month in the refrigerator.

Makes 2 quarts

| CALORIES per 1/3 cup | 115 |
|---|---|
| 68% Carbohydrate | 22 g |
| 5% Protein | 2 g |
| 27% Fat | 4 g |
| CALCIUM | 26 mg |
| IRON | 5 mg |
| SODIUM | 3 mg |

## ORANGE REFRESHER

*This drink provides just as much calcium as a milkshake, but it has less fat and refined sugar, and more protein, vitamin C and potassium.*

3/4 cup orange juice, preferably freshly squeezed

3 1/2 tablespoons nonfat dry milk

3 ice cubes

Fresh mint sprig for garnish (optional)

Fresh orange slices for garnish (optional)

Place the orange juice, milk and ice cubes in a blender and blend until frothy. Pour the drink into a tall glass and garnish with a mint sprig and orange slices if desired.

Makes 1 serving

| CALORIES | 137 |
|---|---|
| 78% Carbohydrate | 27 g |
| 19% Protein | 7 g |
| 3% Fat | .5 g |
| CALCIUM | 204 mg |
| IRON | .4 mg |
| SODIUM | 84 mg |

## PROP CREDITS

Cover: athletic shirt–Calvin Klein Menswear, Inc., New York City; title page: leotard–Dance France Ltd., Santa Monica, Calif.; page 7: shorts–The Gap, San Francisco, Calif.; page 26: leotard–Dance France Ltd., Santa Monica, Calif.; pages 30-53: unitard–Dance France Ltd., Santa Monica, Calif.; weight bench–The Fitness Depot, New York City; page 54: shirt, shorts–The Gap, San Francisco, Calif.; pages 58-75: athletic shirt–Calvin Klein Menswear, Inc., New York City; sweat pants–The Gap, San Francisco, Calif.; massage table–Abbot Exercise Equipment Corp., New York City; pages 80-81: shoes–Nike, Inc., Beaverton, Ore.; pages 82-83: sweatshirt–The Gap, San Francisco, Calif.; shorts–Naturalife, New York City; shoes–Nautilus Athletic Footwear, Inc., Greenville, S.C.; pages 84-85: cycling shorts–Naturalife, New York City; shoes–Nautilus Athletic Footwear, Inc., Greenville, S.C.; pages 86-87: shirt–The Gap, San Francisco, Calif.; shoes–Nautilus Athletic Footwear, Inc., Greenville, S.C.; pages 88-89: shirt, shoes–Naturalife, New York City; shoes–Nautilus Athletic Footwear, Inc., Greenville, S.C.; pages 90-91: athletic shirt–Calvin Klein Menswear, Inc., New York City; shorts–Sportco, Beaverton, Ore.; shoes–Nike, Inc., Beaverton, Ore.; pages 92-93: swimsuit–The Finals, New York City; pages 94-95: shirt, shorts–Naturalife, New York City; shoes–Nautilus Athletic Footwear, Inc., Greenville, S.C.; page 96: sweat pants–The Gap, San Francisco, Calif.; pages 100-123: leotard, tights–Dance France Ltd., Santa Monica, Calif.; exercise mat–AMF American, Jefferson, Iowa; page 129: milk bottle courtesy of Bonnie Slotnick; page 130: plate–Pottery Barn, New York City; tablecloth–Ad-Hoc Softwares, New York City; page 134: plate–Frank McIntosh at Henri Bendel, New York City; napkin–Pottery Barn, New York City; page 137: plate–Gear, New York City; tablecloth–Ad-Hoc Softwares, New York City; page 139: plate–Gear, New York City; page 140: mason jar–Pottery Barn, New York City.

## ACKNOWLEDGMENTS

Gym and pool locations courtesy of New York University.

All cosmetics and grooming products supplied by Clinique Labs, Inc., New York City.

Off-camera warm-up equipment: rowing machine supplied by Precor USA, Redmond, Wash.; washing machine and dryer supplied by White-Westinghouse, Columbus, Ohio; Tunturi stationary bicycle supplied by Amerec Corp., Bellevue, Wash.

Index prepared by Ian Tucker

Production by Giga Communications

## PHOTOGRAPHY CREDIT

All photographs by Steven Mays, Rebus, Inc.

## ILLUSTRATION CREDITS

All illustrations by David Flaherty except illustrations pages 20-21: Stuart Bragg.

*Time-Life Books Inc. offers a wide range of fine recordings, including a Rock 'N' Roll Era series. For subscription information, call 1-800-445-TIME, or write TIME-LIFE MUSIC, Time & Life Building, Chicago, Illinois, 60611.*

# *Index*